THE NAILS IN DISEASE

THE NAILS
IN DISEASE

THIRD EDITION

PETER D SAMMAN, MA, MD, (Camb), FRCP (Lond)

Physician for Diseases of the Skin, Westminster Hospital
Physician to St John's Hospital for Diseases of the Skin

WILLIAM HEINEMANN MEDICAL BOOKS LTD
23 BEDFORD SQUARE, LONDON WC1B 3HH

LMLMLM J

First published 1965
Second edition 1972
Third edition 1978
Reprinted 1980

ISBN 0 433 29152 4

© *Peter D Samman 1978*

Printed in Great Britain by
Western Printing Services Ltd, Bristol

CONTENTS

Preface to Third Edition

It is gratifying to be asked to prepare a third edition of this work. Although the amount of research on nail disorders is very limited, a fair amount of work has been put into the structure of nails and this is recorded.

A number of new clinical conditions are described but the basic aetiology of these is quite unknown and it may be many years before the cause is revealed. There are several new illustrations, all provided either by the photographic departments of St John's Hospital for Diseases of the Skin or Westminster Hospital. I am greatly indebted to them for these and for the older illustrations which have been used again. I remain indebted to the donors of the few additional illustrations acknowledged in the second edition.

I must again thank numerous colleagues who continue to refer cases of nail dystrophy to me and to the publishers for their cooperation and advice.

P D S

Preface to Second Edition

The first edition of this work was well received and filled a need as a practical guide to nail disorders; it is hoped that this new edition will have an equally wide appeal. There were a few criticisms to the first edition and an attempt has been made to correct these in the second. The format remains the same but the book has been completely revised and brought up to date.

The text has been considerably expanded and a number of dermatological conditions not described in the first edition are now included. These often have nail changes sufficiently characteristic to make inclusion justifiable. Many other dermatological conditions show nail changes occasionally but usually of a nonspecific character. No attempt has been made to draw up a comprehensive list of these. Many new illustrations are included and a few of the less satisfactory ones of the first edition have been omitted or replaced.

Many more references are given in this edition than in the first and for convenience these have been placed at the end of each chapter instead of being grouped together at the end of the book. When preparing a textbook, inevitably one refers to the work of previous authors in the same field and in this respect I must acknowledge with gratitude the work of the late Dr. Pardo-Castello (Diseases of the Nails: Pardo-Castello and Pardo, 3rd Edition, c.c. Thomas 1960). Many additional references to earlier reports may be found in that volume.

The two appendices give a list of terms used to describe nail disorders and tables to show the relative frequency of nail conditions as seen by the author.

Most of the illustrations (old and new) were provided by the Photographic Departments of Westminster Hospital and St. John's Hospital for Diseases of the Skin and without their help this work would have been impossible. I am immensely indebted to them. Figures 77 and 87 (both new) were provided by Dr. J. Overton, Figs. 75 and 76 by Dr. Ian Martin-Scott, Fig. 66 by Dr. W. B. McKenna, Fig. 68 by Dr. R. J. Cairns and Fig. 136 by Dr. J. L. Franklin. I am very grateful to each of these.

I should again like to accord my appreciation to numerous colleagues who continue to refer cases of nail dystrophy to me and to the publishers for their co-operation and advice.

London, 1972   P.D.S.

LIST OF COLOUR PLATES

Chapter 1

Anatomy and Physiology

The chief function of the nail in man is that of protection. It protects the delicate terminal phalanx and greatly helps in the appreciation of fine touch and aids in picking up small objects. It is also, of course, used for scratching. A finger deprived of its nail is considerably less valuable than one possessing a nail and

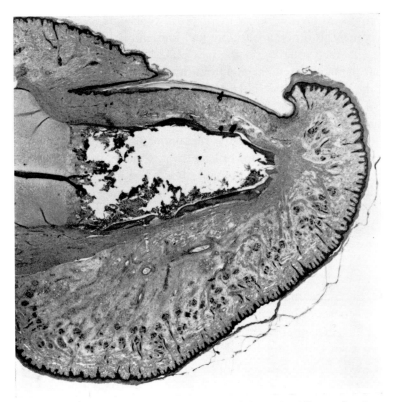

Fig. 1 Longitudinal section through the distal phalanx of a full term foetal toe (photomicrograph)

even the loss of a toe nail is the cause of some hardship. The main reason for complaint in nail deformities is however cosmetic. The nail is greatly modified in some mammals e.g. as a point of loco-motion—the hoof, or as a prehensile organ—the claw.

The nail plate consists of hard keratin and is derived from an invagination of epidermis situated on the dorsum of the terminal phalanx. This invagination is first visible in the 9 week embryo and the formation of the nail is virtually complete by the 20th week (Zaias, 1963). A longitudinal section through the distal phalanx of a full term fetal toe is shown in Fig. 1.

The nail fold consists of a roof, a floor and lateral walls, whilst the nail bed represents that part of the dorsum of the terminal phalanx which lies below the exposed nail plate. There is some argument as to the area of the nail fold and nail bed which takes part in the formation of the nail plate. It is generally accepted that the nail plate is formed from the matrix. The matrix consists of the floor of the nail fold extending from the junction of floor and roof posteriorly to the anterior end of the lunula in front. The latter may or may not be visible but can usually be seen on the thumbs. It is paler than the remainder of the nail plate. It is probable that a small part of the roof of the nail fold also takes part in the formation of the nail plate. The upper surface of the nail is formed from the most proximal portion of the matrix (including the roof of the nail fold when this contributes to the plate) whilst the lower surface is formed from the area close to the distal edge of the lunula. The nail bed itself is generally considered to take no part in the formation of the nail plate (Fig. 2(*a*)). This view was supported by Zaias and Alverez (1968) in experiments on the squirrel monkey, a primate with a flat nail very similar to that of man. They showed by autoradiographic studies following the injection of tritiated glycine either intraperitoneally or into the tissues around the nail that the matrix alone supplied material to the nail plate. Later similar experiments (Norton, 1971) on human volunteers however showed that there was some activity in the nail bed and so the formation of the nail in the squirrel monkey is somewhat different from that in humans.

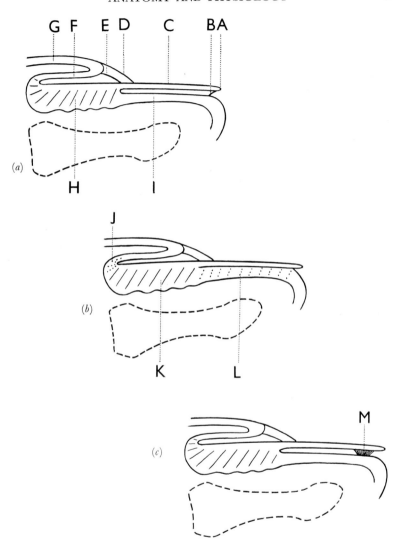

Fig. 2 Nail formation—diagrammatic—antero-posterior section

a. Traditional theory
b. Theory of Lewis
c. Theory of Boas
A. Free margin of nail
B. Hyponychium
C. Nail plate
D. Cuticle
E. Eponychium

F. Roof of nail fold
G. Skin overlying posterior nail fold
H. Matrix
I. Nail bed
J. Matrix of dorsal nail
K. Matrix of intermediate nail
L. Matrix of ventral nail
M. Solenhorn

Barton Lewis (1954) put forward the view that the nail is formed in three layers which he calls dorsal, intermediate and ventral nails. The intermediate nail is the main portion and is derived from the greater part of the (conventional) matrix; the dorsal nail is derived from the roof and a small portion of floor of the nail fold, whilst the ventral nail arises from the nail bed distal to the lunula (Fig. 2 (b)). The lateral walls of the nail fold also contribute material to the nail plate. Although there is some doubt on the validity of Lewis' theory there is no doubt that under pathological conditions material may at times be added to the nail plate from a large part of the nail bed and this fact is of importance in the interpretation of some nail disorders. Histochemical studies show that the material of the upper surface and that of the lower surface of the nail plate stains differently from the true hard keratin of the greater part of the nail (Achten 1963; Jarrett and Spearman, 1966). The firm adhesion of the nail plate to the nail bed, although in part accounted for by corrugations on the under surface of the nail plate fitting into similar corrugations on the nail bed, strongly suggests that the nail bed does contribute to the nail plate. The question whether this material should be accepted as nail keratin is problematical. Achten (1972) does not consider it to be true nail. These two opposing views of nail formation are illustrated diagrammatically in Figs. 2 (a) and (b).

In mammals possessing a claw the matrix consists of two portions, one giving rise to the superficial stratum and the other to the deep stratum of the claw (Fig. 3). In the flat nail of most primates the deep stratum is lost and only the superficial stratum remains (Le Gros Clark, 1959). The deep stratum, if it persisted, would correspond approximately to Lewis' ventral nail.

Pinkus (1927) quotes Boas (1894) in describing the nail bed as consisting of three parts. (1) The proximal part extending as far forward as the distal margin of the lunula which is the nail forming or fertile part of the nail bed. (2) The part on which the nail lies and takes no part in the formation of the nail and is the sterile part of the nail bed. It extends from the distal margin of the lunula to the line where the anterior edge of the nail separates from the bed, the yellow line also known as the onychodermal band (Terry, 1955). (3) The 'sole horn' (sohlenhorn) which again brings horny substance to the nail but does not form actual nail. This is the anterior fertile part or terminal matrix (Fig. 2 (*c*)). It is perhaps this 'sole horn' which can become more extensive under

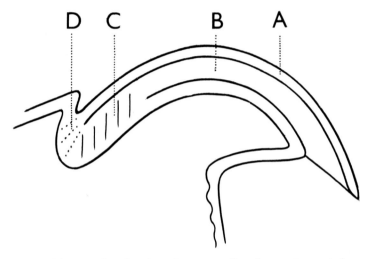

Fig. 3 Diagram of section through a mammalian claw—antero-posterior
(Based on Clark)

A.	Superficial stratum	C.	Terminal matrix
B.	Deep stratum	D.	Basal matrix

pathological conditions, and may be the only vestige of the deep stratum (of a claw) normally present in humans. It is certainly not always present, even as a vestige, but is probably more often present on the toes than on the fingers. Its presence probably accounts for the appearance of spicules of nail which may form towards the tip of the digit after attempts at permanent ablation of the nail and matrix.

The author believes that all three modes of nail formation can occur in normal subjects but that participation of much of the nail bed below the exposed nail is commoner in pathological conditions than in health.

Although the nail bed may at times take no part in the formation of the nail plate it is firmly attached to the nail, and if the
nail is torn off, the epidermis of the nail bed remains attached to
the nail. It is probable that the epidermis of the nail bed moves
forward with the growth of the nail. This epidermis is sometimes
called the hyponychium. The term hyponychium is at times

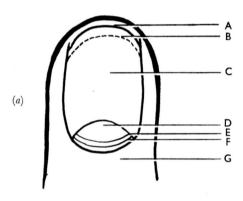

(a)

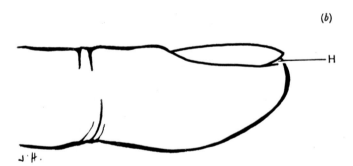

(b)

Fig. 4 Principal features of the nail (*a*) from above and (*b*) from the side
(Diagram based on Pinkus 1927)

A.	Free margin of nail	E.	Cuticle
B.	Point of separation of nail from bed—	F.	Eponychium
	'yellow line' or onychodermal band	G.	Skin overlying posterior nail fold
C.	Nail plate	H.	Area of 'sole horn'
D.	Lunula		

however used in a more restrictive sense to describe a forward extension of the epidermis of the floor of the nail fold on to the under surface of the nail. Used in this way the term is more comparable with the use of the term eponychium (see below).

The cuticle is an extension of the epidermis (usually only the horny layer) of the smooth skin of the dorsum of the finger on to the nail plate, and it may extend quite a long way on to the nail (Figs. 2 and 4). If the cuticle is pushed back too roughly and cut, which often occurs if manicure is done clumsily, it is destroyed and this opens up the space between the nail plate and the roof of the nail fold.

The eponychium is an anterior extension of the roof of the nail fold on to the nail plate and also consists only of epidermis (Figs. 2 and 4). It is of little importance clinically.

In the adult finger about a third of the nail plate is covered by the posterior fold and the matrix entends for 1 to 2 mm beyond the apparent commencement of the nail plate because the nail plate is extremely thin at its point of origin. The space between the matrix and the upper surface of the distal phalanx is very small.

The histology of the nail bed is similar to that of skin except that the epidermal layer is devoid of stratum lucidum and stratum granulosum and there are no secretory or pilosebaceous adnexae. The dermis of the nail bed is arranged in longitudinal grooves and ridges. The rete ridges (of the epidermis) are thin and project into the grooves of the dermis. The epidermis of the nail matrix is thick and passes gradually into the substance of the nail plate. The plate is formed by a series of changes similar to keratinisation of the epidermis namely swelling of the cells followed by nucleolysis and subsequent shrinkage (Lewin *et al.*, 1972).

The significance of the lunula is discussed by Burrows (1917). He mentions a number of theories but believes the pale colour is due to looseness of the nail in this region owing to the curious distribution of fibrous tissue beneath it. This however is not the whole explanation because the area of the lunula remains visible on the nail plate after avulsion of the nail whilst the area still remains visible on the nail bed. Both nail and nail bed must therefore contribute to the appearance. It is probably due to a combination of incomplete keratinization in the nail plate and looseness of connective tissue in the nail bed (Lewin, 1965).

Blood Supply

The nail matrix and nail bed are richly supplied with blood. The arterial supply originates from two main arterial arches lying below the nail plate. The arteries forming these arches are branches of the digital arteries after they reach the pulp space of the terminal phalanx. The two digital arteries form a cruciate anastomosis in the pulp space and from the point of union branches arise and pass dorsally from the palmar space around the thin waist of the distal phalanx (Plate II). In this area they are in a confined space bounded medially by the bone and laterally by a dense ligament which extends from the ungual process anteriorly to the lateral ligament of the distal interphalangeal joint behind (Flint, 1955). On emerging from the space the artery divides, one branch anastomosing with its fellow of the opposite side to form a

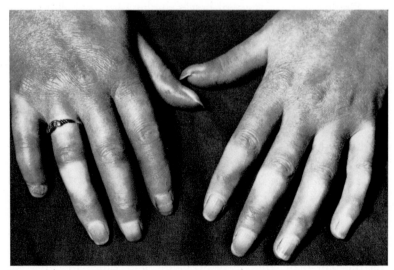

Fig. 5 Progressive scleroderma (acrosclerosis) showing preservation of thumb nails in the presence of pulp atrophy. Partial destruction of nail of right little finger

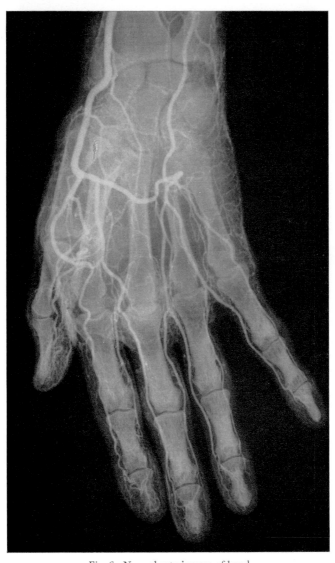

Fig. 6 Normal arteriogram of hand

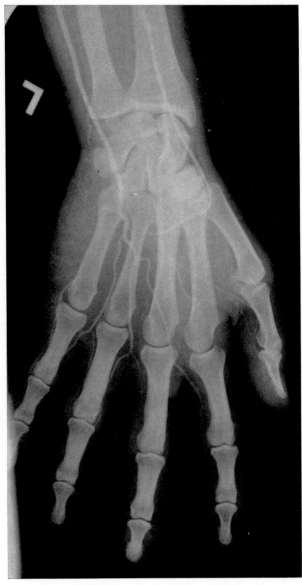

Fig. 7 Arteriogram showing spasm of digital vessels

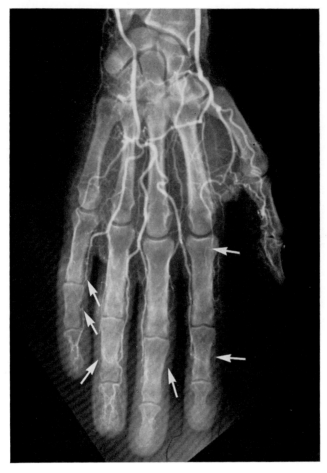

Fig. 8 Arteriogram showing organic blockage of many digital vessels

distal arcade and the other to form a proximal arcade. The proximal arcade also receives a contribution from the middle segment of the finger as a vessel passing dorsally over the distal interphalangeal joint (Flint, 1955; Plate II). This vessel takes part in the formation of a superficial arcade which supplies blood to the skin at the nail base as well as branches to the proximal

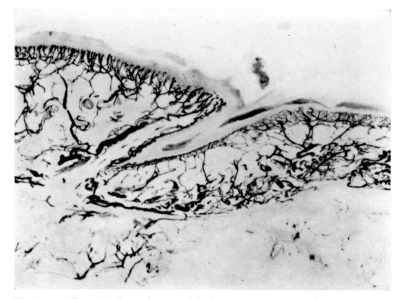

Fig. 9 Capillary blood supply to nail fold. Thick section, blood vessels injected antero-posterior

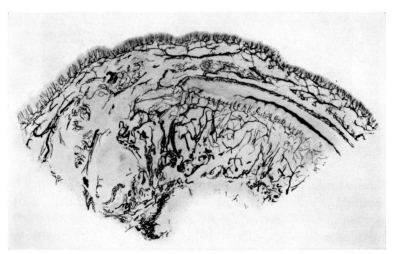

Fig. 10 Same as *Fig. 9* Transverse section mid-way between tip of nail fold and cuticle

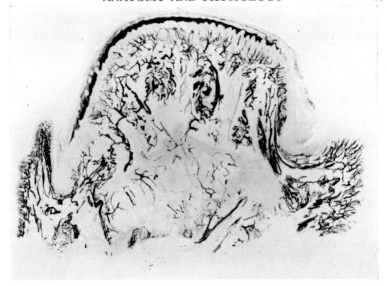

Fig. 11 Capillary blood supply to nail bed. Thick section, blood vessels injected—
transverse

arcade. This accessory blood supply is probably responsible for
allowing the nail to grow normally when the main digital vessels
have been obliterated in the pulp space as may occur in scleroderma of the progressive type (Fig. 5) or in pulp space infections.
A normal arteriogram (Fig. 6) shows the plentiful blood supply to
the pulp. For comparison arteriograms showing spasm (Fig. 7)
and arterial blockage (Fig. 8) are shown.

The capillary blood supply to the tissues around the nail is
abundant. Similar to the capillary loop system of the skin, there
exists a capillary loop system supplying the whole of the nail fold
(Figs. 9, 10 and 11). In a small area beneath the lunula the loop
system was ill defined in specimens examined by the author, but
this may have been the result of incomplete filling.

The nail bed is also richly supplied with glomus bodies which
are probably concerned in the regulation of the blood supply to
the extremities in cold weather. There is also a very rich supply
of lymphatic vessels.

Although the normal blood supply to the nail is so good, defective peripheral circulation is one of the major causes of nail deformities. This is probably largely due to the ease with which the digital arteries go into spasm.

Nail Growth

Unlike hairs, nail growth is continuous throughout life and ceases at death. The apparent continuing growth for 2 or 3 days after death is probably due to shrinkage of the soft tissues around the nail. Although the rate of growth varies greatly from person to person, it is fairly constant in any one individual, but is rather more rapid in youth than in old age. This is well shown by Hamilton *et al.* (1955) who also show that the nails gradually thicken with age. The average rate of growth of finger nails varies between 0.5 and 1.2 mm per week (Hillman, 1955). The author has measured the rate of growth in many nail disorders and can confirm this finding. Bean (1933, 1963, 1968 and 1974) has recorded personal observations on the growth of his own thumb nail continuously over periods of 10, 20, 25 and 30 years. He noted a decided slowing during the second period and a levelling out later. The rate of growth varies slightly from finger to finger as shown by Dawber (1970). This work confirmed the earlier observations of Le Gros Clark and Buxton (1958). Generally it may be said that the longer the finger the more rapid the nail growth, therefore the middle finger has the most rapid growth followed by index and ring finger, whilst the thumb and little finger nails have the slowest rate. Nails on the right hand grow slightly quicker than those on the left. Many measurements are required to show up these small but significant differences. Dawber (1970) has also shown that in psoriasis apparently normal nails grow significantly faster (taken as a group) than the corresponding nails of normal subjects. Nails showing pitting grow even faster than the apparently normal nails. Owing to the wide range of normal growth rate groups of patients rather than individuals have to be considered in these measurements. A similar observation has been made for nails showing idiopathic onycholysis where the rate of growth may be much higher than normal (Dawber *et al.*, 1971). Nail growth may also be speeded up in the presence of inflammatory change around the nail and in the bullous form of congenital ichthyosiform erythroderma. Growth rate may be temporarily depressed in many general medical illnesses or generalised skin complaints. Sibinga (1959) observed that measles constantly depressed the rate of nail growth in young children for a short time. Both Bean and Sibinga also noted that a severe attack of mumps caused a temporary slowing of nail growth. There is one condition described on p. 119 under the heading of 'yellow nail syndrome' in which the rate of growth is constantly very slow. The average length of time taken for a finger nail to grow from the matrix to the free edge is about $5\frac{1}{2}$ months. Toe nails grow at about $\frac{1}{2}$ to $\frac{1}{3}$ the rate of finger nails and replacement takes 12–18 months. Kligman (1961) wondered why nails should grow forward rather than up, and concluded that it is due to pressure exerted by the posterior nail fold. If a portion of nail matrix is auto-grafted on to skin away from the nail fold it will produce a nail but one which projects straight upwards. Hashimoto *et al.* (1966) believe that forward growth is the result of all matrix cells being orientated in a forward direction.

Structure of Nail

Not a great deal of work has been done on the structure of nail, much less than on wool with its great commercial value. The nail plate is curved in both directions (antero-posterior and lateral) giving it greater strength. Light microscopic studies show it to be made up of layers of cells deprived of nuclei and flattened in the plane of the nail surface. Forslind (1970) has studied nails with the electronmicroscope and with X-ray diffraction techniques and considers their hardness to be due to the cell arrangement and cell adhesion and the ultrastructural arrangement of keratin fibrils. The latter are intercellular and are mainly orientated parallel to the nail surface from side to side. These findings were confirmed in scanning electron microscopic studies (Forslind and Thyresson, 1975). Keratin itself is a protein containing a high proportion of sulphur mainly in the form of cystine and in nail constitutes 9.4% by weight. There is a natural line of cleavage between dorsal and intermediate nails. The dorsal nail is much harder than the intermediate but the latter is more pliable and therefore less brittle.

Forslind states that the calcium content of nail is very low and in no case that he studied did it constitute more than 2 parts per 1000 by weight. It is suggested that most of this calcium is in the upper surface of the nail plate and is probably derived from the environment (soap etc.) rather than from within. Robson and Brooks (1974) studied the distribution of calcium in finger nails from healthy and malnourished children and found that in kwashiorkor it was not possible to distinguish between dorsal, intermediate or ventral portions in respect of calcium content.

Nitrogen, calcium and a number of other elements in nail were estimated by Veller (1970) in an attempt to assess whether there was any appreciable nutritional loss resulting from the constant growth and clipping of nails. The loss was shown to be negligible.

Harrison and Clemena (1972) have shown that by spark source mass spectometry it is possible to estimate the quantity of many trace elements in human finger nail clippings.

References

Achten, G (1963) L'Ongle Normal et Pathologique. *Dermatologica* **126** 229

Achten, G (1972) Histologie Ungueale. *Bull. Dell'istituto Derm. S. Gall.* **8** 3

Bean, W B (1953) A Note on Finger Nail Growth. *J. invest. Derm.* **20** 27

Bean, W B (1963) Nail Growth. *Arch. intern. Med.* **111** 476

Bean, W B (1968) Nail Growth. *Arch. intern. Med.* **122** 359

Bean, W B (1974) Nail Growth 30 years of observation. *Arch. intern. Med.* **134** 497

Boas, I E U (1894) Zur Morphologie der Wirbeltirkralle Morphol. *Jb. Bd.* 21, p. 281

Burrows, M T (1917) The Significance of the Lunula of the Nail. *Anat. Rec.* **12** 161

Clark, W E Le Gros (1959) The Antecedents of Man. Edinburgh.

Clark, W E Le Gros and Buxton, L H D (1938) Studies in Nail Growth. *Brit. J. Derm.* **50** 221

Dawber, R (1970) Finger Nail Growth in Normal and Psoriatic Subjects. *Brit. J. Derm.* **82** 454

Dawber, R, Samman, P D and Bottoms, E (1971) Nail Growth in Idiopathic and Psoriatic Onycholysis, *Brit. J. Derm.* **85** 558

Flint, M H (1955) Some Observations on the Vascular Supply of the Nail Bed and Terminal Segments of the Finger. *Brit. J. Plast. Surg.* **8** 186

Forslind, B (1970) Biophysical Studies of the Normal Nail. *Acta. dermvener (Stockholm)* **50** 161

Forslind, B and Thyresson, N (1975) On the Structure of the Normal Nail. A Scanning Electon Miscroscope Study. *Arch. Derm. Forsche.* **251** 199

Hamilton, J B, Terada, H and Mestler, G E (1955) Studies of Growth Throughout the Life Span in Japanese; Growth and Size of Nails and their Relationship to Age, Sex, Heredity and other factors. *J. Geront.* **10** 401

Harrison, W W and Clemena, G G (1972) Survey analysis of trace elements in human finger nails by spark source mass spectrometry. *Clin. Chim. Acta.* **36** 485

Hashimoto, K, Gross, B G, Nelson, R and Lever, W F (1966) The Ultra-Structure of the Skin of Human Embryos III. The Formation of the Nail in 16–18 weeks old Embryos. *J. invest. Derm.* **17** 205

Jarrett, A and Spearman, R I C (1966) Histochemistry of the Human Nail. *Arch. Derm.* **94** 652

Kligman, A M (1961) Why do Nails grow out instead of up? *Arch. Derm.* **84** 313

Lewin, K (1965) The Normal Finger Nail. *Brit. J. Derm.* **77** 421

Lewin, K, De Wit, S and Ferrington, R A (1972) Pathology of the finger nail in psoriasis. *Brit. J. Derm.* **86** 555

Lewis, B L (1954) Microscopic Studies of Foetal and Mature Nail and Surrounding Soft Tissue. *Arch. Derm.* **70** 732

Norton, L A (1971) Incorporation of the thymidine-methyl H³ and glycine 2 H³ in the nail matrix and bed of humans. *J. invest. Derm.* **56** 61

Pinkus, F (1927) in Jadassohn, J *Handbuck der Haut und Geschlechtskrankeiten*, 1/1 Julius Springer, Berlin, pp. 267–289

Robson, J R K and Brooks, G J (1974) The distribution of calcium in Finger Nails from Healthy and Malnourished children. *Clin. Chim. Acta.* **55** 255

Samman, P D (1959) The Human Toe Nail. Its Genesis and Blood Supply. *Brit. J. Derm.* **71** 296

Sibinga, M S (1959) Observations on Growth of Finger Nails in Health and Disease. *Pediatrics* **24** 225

Terry, R B (1955) The Onychodermal Band in Health and Disease. *Lancet* **i** 179

Vellar, O D (1970) Composition of human nail substance. *Am. J. Clin. Nutrition* **23** 1272

Zaias, N (1963) Embryology of the Human Nail. *Arch. Derm.* **87** 37

Zaias, N and Alvarez, J (1968) The Formation of the Primate Nail Plate. An Autoradiographic Study in the Squirrel Monkey. *J. invest. Derm.* **57** 120

Chapter 2

Principal Nail Symptoms

This chapter is inserted as an aid to diagnosis. The nails can react in relatively few ways so that the same symptoms occur in several different conditions.

The pathological processes responsible for most nail changes are unknown. This is due largely to the difficulty in processing the nails and surrounding structures for microscopical examination. It is very difficult to obtain adequate longitudinal sections through the nail, bed and matrix, even post-mortem so that with few exceptions biopsies from living subjects are disappointing. Zaias (1967) has however described a method of taking longitudinal biopsies through the nail which he claims does not leave a permanent split in the nail. With Alvarez (1967) he described a method of processing a nail biopsy for section. Achten (1972) showed that histological examination of nail clippings may be helpful.

Absence

Anonychia—absence of the nail from birth is considered in Chapter 12 p. 171. It may also occur in the nail patella syndrome, p. 167.

Brittleness

Brittle nails are very common and little is known of the basic pathology. Causes may be local or general. Of the systemic causes impaired peripheral circulation (p. 104) and iron deficiency anaemia are the most frequent. Among local causes constant immersion of the hands in water especially if alkaline is the chief offender (Silver and Chiego, 1940). Diffuse alopecia associated with brittle nails has been recorded as a manifestation of an enzyme disturbance of arginine metabolism (Shelley and Rawnsley, 1956). In many cases the cause is quite obscure. The treatment of brittle nails is considered on p. 101.

Discoloration

The colour of the nail may be altered in many ways and these may be grouped as shown below.

(a) Staining from external causes: dyes encountered at work or in other ways including hair dyes, nicotine, medicaments applied by the patient to himself or others (mercury, vioform, dithranol, resorcin, picric acid, etc.) and tints leaking out of nail varnish (p. 139). Pseudomonas aeruginosa infection under or adjacent to the nail will stain the nail black or blue.

(b) Abnormal formation of the nail: severe psoriasis is the most important condition under this heading. Much less common are acrodermatitis continua, pityriasis rubra pilaris, pachyonychia congenita, alopecia areata and Darier's disease.

(c) Degenerative changes occurring in a nail after formation: yellow nail syndrome, congenital ectodermal defect and in old age. All are due to the slow growth of the nail.

(d) Partial destruction after formation: fungal and candidal infections often cause a brownish discoloration of the nail but occasionally whiten the nail. Brown or black discoloration of the nail edge is common in chronic paronychia.

(e) Incorporation of a stain in the nail during formation: a yellow colour may develop in all nails during prolonged tetracycline administration.

(f) Miscellaneous causes: drugs may alter the colour of the nails in other ways (p. 99). Black streaks are very common in the nails of coloured races and are of little or no significance (p. 128). A single black streak in a white person may be due to a junctional naevus in the nail matrix (p. 156). Multiple pigment streaks may occur in Addison's disease (Allenby and Snell, 1966). Subcutaneous haemorrhage is the commonest cause of blackening of part of a nail. The half moons may become blue in Kinnier Wilson's disease or red in cardiac failure.

(g) Leukonychia and whitening due to changes in the nail bed are considered on pp. 93 and 117.

Haemorrhage

Subungual haematomata are almost always due to trauma. Splinter haemorrhages below the nails are discussed on p. 121. In addition to general medical disorders they are also found in psoriasis, dermatitis and fungous infections.

Hypertrophy

Probably the great majority of hypertrophied nails are the result of trauma but they also occur as developmental anomalies in pachyonychia congenita and ectodermal defects. The little toe nail is often thickened as an isolated phenomenon and closely resembles a claw. Sometimes this change is associated with hyperkeratosis of the feet or elsewhere. Touraine and Soulignac (1937) described a case where all toe nails were thickened in association with other developmental anomalies. Stauffer (1942) described a number of cases of thickening of the great toe nails. These might be shed and replaced by a nail which again hypertrophied. Some patients also had sebaceous cysts.

Other causes of nail hypertrophy are psoriasis, fungal infections, pityriasis rubra pilaris and Darier's disease.

Koilonychia

Most characteristically seen as a symptom of iron deficiency anaemia, koilonychia is also found as a congenital anomaly, as a temporary disorder in young children, and in association with thinning of the nail plate from any cause. Both halves of a split nail in the nail patella syndrome may show koilonychia. In some cases no cause can be found.

Onycholysis
(Separation of the nail from its bed)

This is one of the commonest of nail symptoms. It is found as part of the symptomatology of psoriasis, fungous infections, dermatitis of the finger tips and rarely in drug eruptions. It is also found in defective peripheral circulation, the yellow nail syndrome, shell nail syndrome, congenital ectodermal defect, in thyroid disorders and in association with hyperhidrosis. Trauma of various kinds may initiate or aggravate the condition but some cases appear to be idiopathic and these are discussed on p. 88. It is occasionally met with as an occupational disease e.g. in poultry pluckers (Forck and Kastner, 1967).

Pitting

Psoriasis is the commonest cause of nail pitting but pits are also found in dermatitis, alopecia areata and funguous infection. Minor degrees of pitting are common in persons with otherwise healthy nails and with no other skin complaints.

Pterygium Formation

This is a progressive complaint usually starting on one nail and extending to others. The cuticle appears to grow forward on the

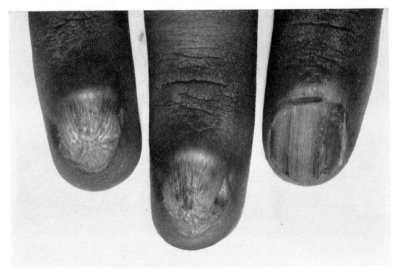

Fig. 12 Pterygium formation. Just starting on ring finger and complete on index and middle fingers

nail plate and the nail is split into two portions which gradually get smaller as the pterygium widens. It may extend to complete loss of the nail or small remnants may remain. Histologically it can be seen to result from fusion of the epidermis of the dorsal nail fold to the nail bed including the matrix. It occurs as a result of impaired peripheral circulation and in severe lichen planus. In a few cases however no cause can be found (Fig. 12) including those occurring in idiopathic atrophy of the nail (p. 96).

Shedding

Nail loss may be the result of loosening at the base (onychomadesis) or separation from the nail bed (onycholysis) extending until the whole nail becomes loose and comes away completely. Nail loss should further be divided into loss without and loss with scarring.

Loss without Scarring

Periodic shedding is an uncommon congenital anomaly discussed on p. 174. Loss of one or two nails especially the great toe nails is not uncommon and although no cause can normally be found it is probably due to minor trauma in most cases. The nail will often be shed following a subungual haematoma. Severe onycholysis from any cause may progress to temporary nail loss. This is especially characteristic of the yellow nail syndrome (p. 119). The nails are occasionally shed after severe illness (see under Beau's lines p. 112) or as a reaction to drugs (p. 98).

Loss with Scarring

This is the most serious nail symptom. It may occasionally follow trauma, defective peripheral circulation, lichen planus, epidermolysis bullosa and bullous drug eruptions. It may occur as part of some congenital anomalies and may be the end result of pterygium formation. Although scarring is present, small portions of nail may remain or regrow.

PLATE I

[a] Psoriasis
(gross changes)

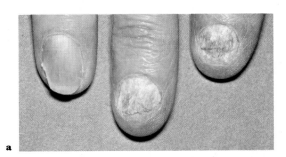

[b] Tinea unguium

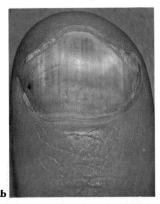

[c] Candidiasis
of nail plates

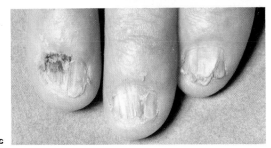

[d] Scopulariopsis
brevicaulis
infection of nails

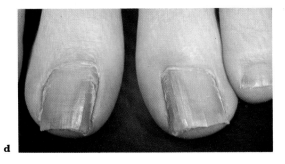

PLATE II

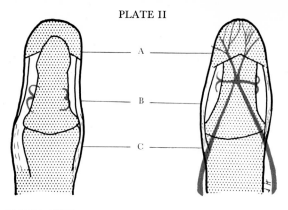

DORSAL VIEW   PALMAR VIEW

a

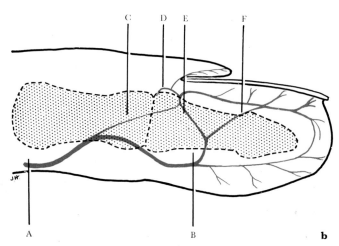

b

[**a**] Diagram of main arterial blood supply to the nail and nail bed from above and below. Based on Flint (1955)
A Ungual spine
B Interosseous ligament
C Collateral ligament

[**b**] Diagram of main arterial supply to the nail and nail bed—lateral view. Based on Flint (1955)
A Digital artery
B Branch of digital artery arising in pulp space
C Branch of digital artery arising in middle segment of finger and reaching nail area without passing through pulp space
D Superficial arcade
E Subdivision of B to form proximal arcade
F Subdivision of B to form distal arcade

Splitting

Splitting into layers is discussed on p. 136. Splitting longitudinally may be the result of trauma and may be temporary or permanent. Excessively ridged nails (see below) are liable to split along the ridges. Thin nails and brittle nails are also liable to split. Some affected nails in the nail patella syndrome may show a single longitudinal split (p. 167).

Striations

Longitudinal striations are common in health but are usually of minor degree in young persons, becoming more prominent in old age. Exaggeration of the striations may occur in lichen planus, in Darier's disease, in association with defective peripheral circulation and as a developmental anomaly. They are also said to occur more often in patients with rheumatoid arthritis than in normal subjects when the striations may be accompanied by beading.

A single depression through the length of the nail may be due to median dystrophy (p. 90), habit tic (p. 133), or a mucous cyst (p. 154).

Transverse striations of minor degree and regular in appearance may occur as a developmental anomaly and they have also been attributed to difference in the rate of growth of the nail at or near the menstrual period compared with other times. Gross irregular cross striations are found in dermatitis. Gross striations also occur as a result of trauma from excess manicuring or a habit tic. A single depression across a nail may be a Beau's line (p. 112).

Thinning

Thinning of the nail plate is seen in association with defective peripheral circulation, lichen planus, epidermolysis bullosa and iron deficiency anaemia. In many cases however no cause is apparent.

24 THE NAILS IN DISEASE

References

Achten, G (1972) Histologie ungueale. *Bull. Dell-istuto Derm. S. Gall.* **8** 3

Allenby, C F and Snell, F H (1966). Longitudinal pigmentation of the nails in Addison's disease. *Br. med. J.* **1** 1582

Alvarez, R and Zaias, N (1967) A modified polyethylene glycol-pyroxylin embedding method. *J. invest. Derm.* **49** 409

Forck, G and Kastner, H (1967) Charakteristische Onycholysis Traumatica bei Fliehbandarbeiter in Geflugelschlacterei. *Der Hautarzt* **18** 85

Shelley, W B and Rawnsley, H M (1965) Aminogenic alopecia. Loss of hair associated with Argininosuccinic aciduria. *Lancet,* **ii** 1327

Silver, H and Chiego, B (1940). Nails and Nail Changes. Brittleness of nails (Fragilitas Unguium). *J. invest. Derm.* **3** 357

Stauffer, J and Simmons, J (1942) Hyperkeratosis of the large toe-nails and sebaceous cysts. *J. Hered.* **33** 285

Touraine, A et Soulignac, M (1937). Onychogryphose Congénitale généralisée des orteils. *Bull. Soc. fr. Derm. Syph.* **44** 305

Zaias, N (1967) The longitudinal nail biopsy. *J. invest. Derm.* **49** 406

Chapter 3

Psoriasis

Psoriasis is one of the commonest skin diseases and the nails are involved in a high proportion of cases. In Crawford's series (Crawford, 1938) almost 50% of cases had nail involvement. If only a single close inspection is made about 25% of cases will show nail involvement but over a lifetime the incidence must be nearer 80–90%. Finger nails are said to be involved more often than toe nails (Zaias, 1969) but this may be apparent rather than real as toe nail involvement is seldom a cause for complaint. The nails may be involved in the complete absence of psoriasis elsewhere and many of the worst cases of nail involvement show only minimal psoriasis elsewhere. These minimal changes are most likely to be found in the scalp or on the genitalia. Psoriasis is thus the most important single cause of nail dystrophy.

The nails are deformed in many ways. The feature most widely recognised is pitting. This may vary from a few isolated pits on one nail (Fig. 13) to uniform pitting of all nails (Fig. 14). The pits are usually small and seldom more than one mm across and quite shallow. Much larger pits and even punched out areas are seen occasionally. The pits are generally found scattered irregularly over a few nails but occasionally are quite regular and form into lines of pits across the nails. As they may also be produced at regular intervals the pits may form into lines in the long axis of the nails also. This type of regular pitting may also be seen occasionally in alopecia areata. Other common causes of irregular pitting of the nails are dermatitis and chronic parony- chia but these conditions can usually be readily distinguished. Pits may however appear without evidence of skin disease, but are normally very insignificant in such cases. Mottling in the half moon (lunula) is often seen in association with pitting in psoriasis

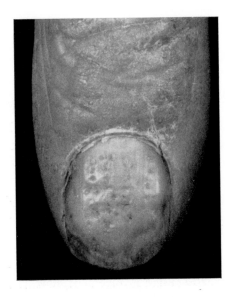

Fig. 13   Psoriasis—pitting

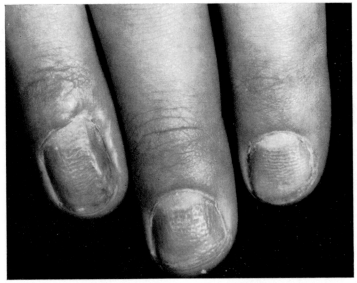

Fig. 14   Psoriasis—uniform pitting

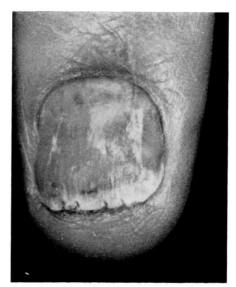

Fig. 15   Psoriasis—pitting with
   mottling in half moon

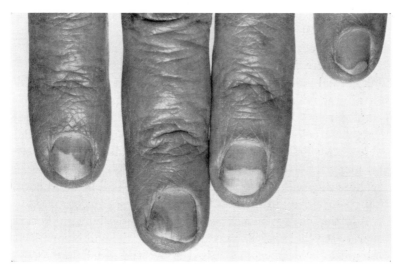

Fig. 16   Psoriasis—onycholysis

(Fig. 15) and sometimes with pitting from other causes e.g. alopecia areata (Fig. 67).

Alkiewiez (1948) showed that the pits are due to retention of nuclei (parakeratosis) in parts of the nail keratin. These areas are weaker than the surrounding normal keratin and may be shed leaving the pits on the nail surface. Zaias (1969) has shown more exactly how this occurs. A scanning electron microscopic study of normal and psoriatic nails (Mauro *et al.*, 1975) has shown that the surface of normal nails is made up of overlapping flat cells with the overlap opposite to the direction of growth. The cell surfaces are generally flat and closely opposed. A few micropits are visible. The pits of psoriatic nails differ from normal nails in that the cells on the surface are smaller and do not have the overlapping pattern. They appear to be heaped up and to be growing in a haphazard way and seem to be crowded together. There are spaces between the poorly interdigitated cells. Numerous micropits are also seen.

Onycholysis, or separation of the nail from its bed is not so well recognised as part of psoriasis but occurs almost as often as pitting. The separation is usually partial and involves one or several nails (Fig. 16). It most commonly starts at the free edge of the nail but may commence in the centre of the nail plate. Onycholysis occurs in many conditions other than psoriasis but in psoriasis there is usually a yellow margin visible between the pink normal nail and the white separated area. If the separation starts in the middle of the nail the yellow margin will form into a complete ring (Fig. 17). Although not pathognomonic of psoriasis this yellow colour is only seen occasionally in lysis from other causes. Onycholysis may come on quite suddenly in psoriasis and many nails may become involved overnight. It is apparent therefore that it is due to an alteration in the nail bed and not to changes occurring in the matrix area.

A further change seen occasionally is apparently a complication of severe onycholysis. The proximal part of the nail bed with the nail still attached becomes raised above the distal part so that the nail is very widely separated and, for comfort, the patient is

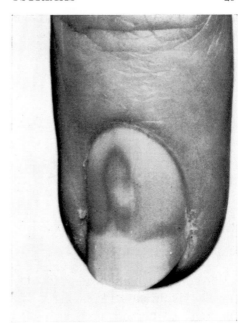

Fig. 17 Psoriasis—onycholysis
starting in centre of nail plate

then forced to cut the nail very short (Figs. 18 and 19). Psoriasis
is probably the most common cause of onycholysis but it may
occur under many other circumstances (p. 20).

The third and most distressing change in the nails seen in
psoriasis is a grosser abnormality of the nail plate. The nail loses

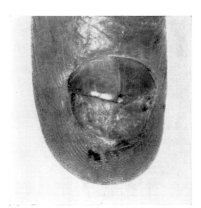

Fig. 18 Psoriasis—onycholysis with wide
separation of nail from its bed

its lustre, becomes opaque, discoloured, irregular and may be thickened. The process may be seen to start as the nail emerges

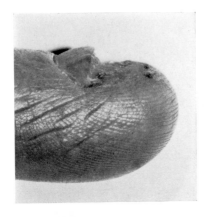

Fig. 19   Psoriasis—same as *Fig. 18* lateral view

from under the cuticle and moves forward as the nail grows to involve the whole nail plate (Fig. 20). One or several nails may be involved but not necessarily all to the same extent. Often

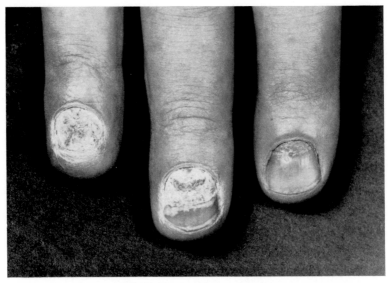

Fig. 20   Psoriasis—gross changes

however by the time the patient reports most nails are totally involved. It is apparent that this type of change is dependent on abnormalities in the matrix area. The deformity is not static but may show constant change, one nail returning to normal whilst others become involved. This changing pattern is seldom seen with other nail disorders (Fig. 21). Zaias (1969) says that the colour change is due to large amounts of a serum-like exudate containing glycoprotein which accumulates in and under the affected nails. He says this glycoprotein is commonly found in inflammatory and eczematous diseases affecting the nail bed but not in fungal infections. Part of the colour change is however due to minute haemorrhages in the nail bed visible through the nail plate.

The only important differential diagnosis in this third type of deformity is fungal or candidal infection of the nail plate. The colour and irregularity may be seen in either and subungual haemorrhages may occur in either. With fungous infections however it is always possible to find the organism in potash preparations and the nail plate is usually softer than in psoriasis. Leyden et al. (1972) describe a method of examining nail shavings and subungual hyperkeratosis to show up parakeratotic cells in psoriasis which they did not find in other nail disorders except for occasional nucleated cells in onychomycosis.

Very seldom are dermatophytes found in association with nail psoriasis although yeasts and bacteria are commonly present in the subungual debris (Zaias, 1969), and it has been pointed out that chronic paronychia (Chapter 5) is commonly found in association with nail psoriasis (Ganor, 1975).

Great thickening of the nail is another less common change in psoriasis. The appearances are similar to those just described except that the nail is greatly thickened by incorporation of much material from the nail bed into the nail (ventral nail). This is more often found in toe than in finger nails. A similar change is found occasionally in Darier's disease and in pachyonychia congenita.

The formation of hard material at the edge of the nail lifting

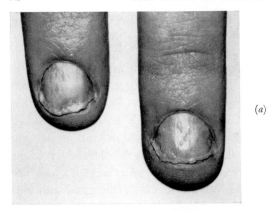

(a)

(b)

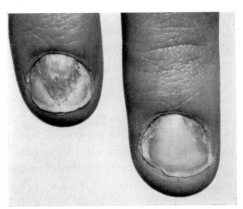

Fig. 21 Psoriasis—to show
    changing pattern
    (a) November 1961
    (b) September 1962
    (c) December 1962

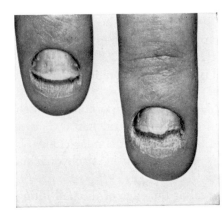

(c)

the nail from its bed and distorting the nail plate is another
feature of psoriasis which may occur in association with, or
independently of the other conditions described. Over curvature
of one or more nails may be seen occasionally (Fig. 22).

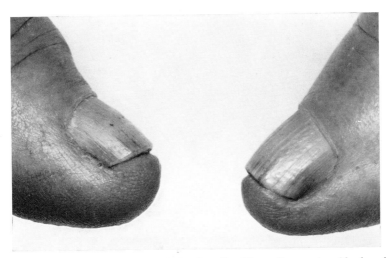

Fig. 22 Psoriasis—overcurvature of thumb nails. The nails are also ridged and
beaded due to ageing (patient aged 83)

Lewin *et al.* (1972) investigated the histological changes in the
nail matrix and nail bed in psoriasis and showed that there was a
metaplastic change in both areas producing a skin-like epithelium
so that the histology resembled that of normal skin.

Arthropathy involving the distal inter-phalangeal joints may
occur with severe nail psoriasis (Fig. 23), but is rare compared
with the number of cases in whom the nails are involved without
arthritis. The arthritis is of a destructive type but is almost certainly not the same as rheumatoid arthritis. X-ray will show the
joint changes and there is often destruction of the distal phalanx.
The Rose–Waaler test is negative.

Treatment of psoriasis of the nails is unsatisfactory. The condition often improves spontaneously and may improve as skin
lesions resolve with or without treatment. Improvement of the
severe type of change will usually occur following injections of

triamcinolone into the matrix area but the improvement is normally short-lived unless the injections are repeated. Needle injections are however painful but the use of the 'Porton gun' (Abell, 1972) or similar apparatus is not recommended owing to

(a)

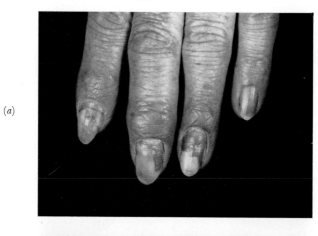

(b)

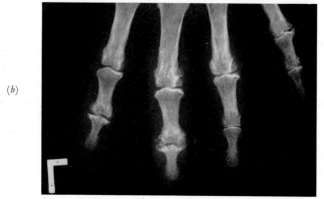

Fig. 23 (*a* and *b*) Psoriasis of nails and arthropathy of distal inter-phalangeal joints

the difficulty in sterilising the apparatus.   It is theoretically possible to transfer a viral infection from one patient to the next with the gun. The application of 0.025% fluocinolone acetonide cream or other fluorinated topical steriod creams under polythene occlusion is worthy of trial. It produces improvement in some cases where the nails are badly affected but must not be repeated indefinitely or atrophy of the soft tissues around the nail will occur. Fredriksson (1974) obtained useful improvement from the topical application of 1% 5 fluorouracil solution without occlusion over a period of 6 months. About 25 ml of the solution was used each month. X-ray therapy will occasionally induce a remission which may last months or years and may therefore be tried if other methods fail. The dose required is 100 rad at 60 or 70 kV repeated at weekly intervals to a total of 400 or 500 rad. The nail beds do not stand a great deal of X-ray therapy so the treatment should not be repeated more than once or twice in the patient's lifetime. Onycholysis is seldom improved by this treatment. In the great majority of cases the best treatment is to reassure the patient in the hope that a spontaneous remission may occur. Intense ultraviolet light has been used successfully by Holti in some cases (p. 109).

Pustular Psoriasis and Acrodermatitis Continua

The nail changes in these conditions are the same as the

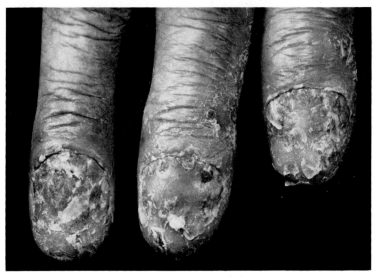

Fig. 24 Pustular psoriasis

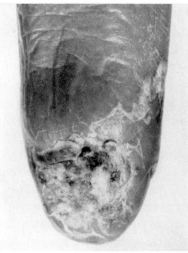

Fig. 25 Acrodermatitis

Fig. 26 Pustular psoriasis before shedding of main part of nails

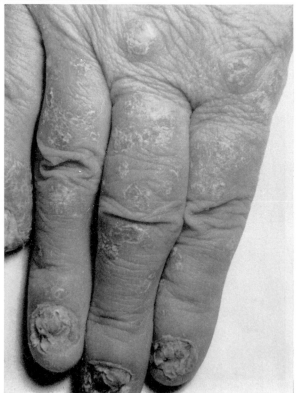

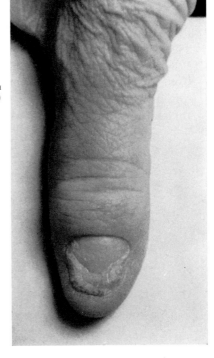

Fig. 27 Same as *Fig. 26* after main portion of nail was shed (see text)

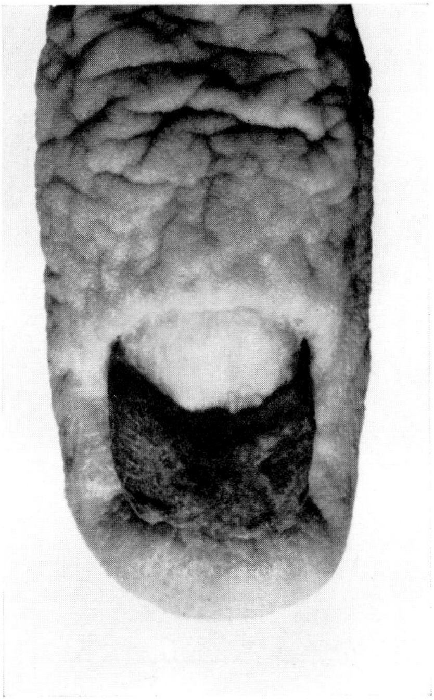

Fig. 28 Same patient as *Fig. 26*— post-mortem

grosser changes in psoriasis and it is probable that they are all variants of the same process (Figs. 24 and 25). Pustules forming under a nail may result in permanent loss of the nail occasionally.

The author has published details of a case of generalised pustular psoriasis (Samman, 1961) in whom all the finger nails were grossly distorted and thickened (Fig. 26). When given treatment with systemic triamcinolone the portion of nail derived from the matrix was shed from each finger and was not replaced so that the nail folds remained empty. Hard keratin arising from the nail bed however remained *in situ* and formed a satisfactory

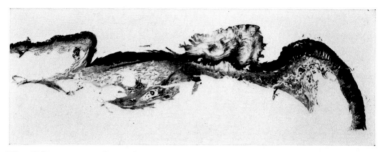

Fig. 29 Low power photomicrograph (× 5)—anteroposterior through nail shown in *Fig. 28*

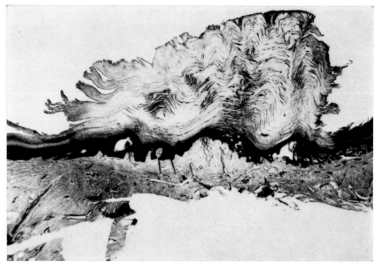

Fig. 30 Higher power photomicrograph (× 17) showing details of " ventral nail " or " sole horn "

nail (Figs. 27 and 28). The portion remaining corresponded to Lewis' ventral nail and appeared quite different from the pseudo-nail which may cover the nail bed if a nail is surgically removed and its matrix destroyed. The ventral nail here was presumably a development from the sole horn (p. 5). The histological appearances of one of these digits is shown in Figs. 29 and 30.

References

Abell, E (1972). Treatment of Psoriatic Nail Dystrophy. *Brit. J. Derm.* **86** 79

Alkiewicz, J (1948) Psoriasis of the Nail. *Brit. J. Derm.* **60** 196

Crawford, G M (1938). Psoriasis of the Nails. *Archs. Derm. Syph.* **38** 583

Fredricksson, T (1974) Topically applied fluorouracil in treatment of psoriatic nails. *Arch. Derm.* **110** 735

Ganor, S (1975) Chronic paronychia and psoriasis. *Brit. J. Derm.* **92** 685

Lewin, K, DeWit, S and Ferrington R A (1972) Pathology of the finger nail in psoriasis. *Br. J. Derm.* **86** 555

Leyden, J J (1972) Exfoliative cytology in the diagnosis of psoriasis of the nails. *Cutis.* **10** 701

Mauro, J, Lumpkin, L R and Danzig, P I (1975) Scanning electron microscopy of psoriatic nail pits. *N.Y. State. J. Med.* **75** 339

Samman, P D (1961) The Ventral Nail. *Arch. Derm. Syph.* **84** 1030

Zaias, N (1969). Psoriasis of the Nail. *Arch. Derm.* **99** 567

Chapter 4

Fungous Infection
(Tinea Unguium: Onychomycosis)

Fungous infections of the nails are very common and the incidence is probably increasing. One or two toe nails are often infected in the presence of tinea pedis and this is often overlooked by the patient who does not seek advice unless many toe nails or the finger nails become infected. There are a number of dermatophytes which will infect the nails and the two most frequently encountered in this country are Trichophyton rubrum and T. mentagrophytes (variety interdigitale). Other fungi found less often are Epidermophyton floccosum, T. sulphureum, T. megninii, T. shoenleinii, T. soudanese, T. violaceum and T. concentricum. The latter two are probably common in countries where these fungi are endemic. Candida albicans may also invade the nail plate and at times produces a deformity very similar to tinea

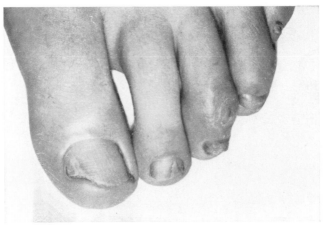

Fig. 31   Early fungous infection of toe nails

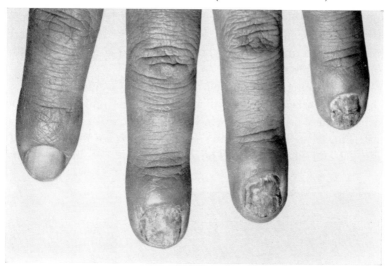

Fig. 32 Extensive fungous infection of finger nails

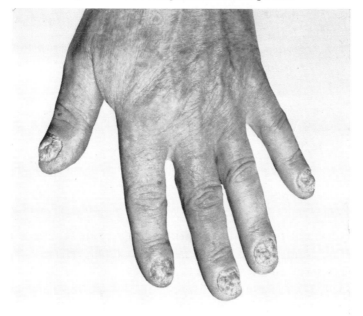

Fig. 33 Fungous infection showing thickening of nail plate

unguium but this is considered separately (Chapter 5). Scopulariopsis brevicaulis infection is usually limited to one or both great toe nails and can often be distinguished clinically from the true dermatophyte infections (p. 48).

Fungous infections will deform the nail in a number of ways. The infection reaches the nail plate from the nail bed and the earliest sign is usually a brownish discoloration at the edge of the nail (Fig. 31). This may later spread to involve the whole nail (Fig. 32 and Plate I (*b*)). The nail bed may become thick and

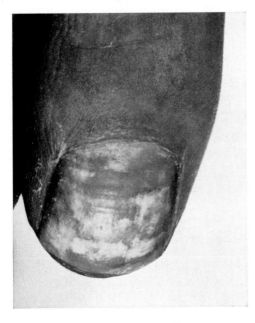

Fig. 34 Fungous infection—
white patches

irregular and the nail itself thickened (Fig. 33). The nail may separate from its bed producing onycholysis. At times white patches form on the nail plate (Fig. 34) and this is often the result of cracks forming and producing air spaces in the plate. The space may later become filled with dirt or bacterial contamination may occur, producing a more discoloured nail (Fig. 35). In T. megninii infections especially, the whole nail plate

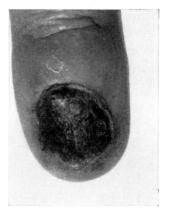

Fig. 35 Fungous infection—gross discoloration

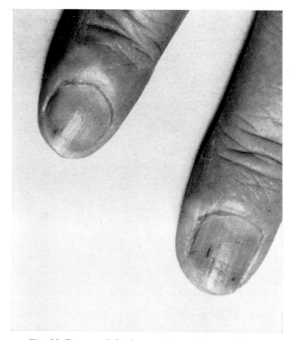

Fig. 36 Fungous infection—subungual haemorrhages

may become white. At times small haemorrhages are visible
through the nail plate (Fig. 36), and these often remain when the

nails are otherwise clinically normal after treatment with griseo-fulvin. Occasionally the nails are shed entirely but more often so much of the infected nail breaks away that only a small remnant remains visible near the cuticle (Fig. 37).

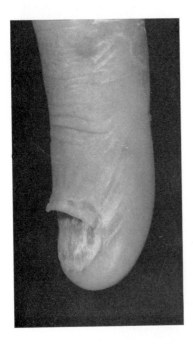

Fig. 37 Fungous infection—nail bed heavily infected; greater part of nail broken away

The diagnosis can usually be suspected by the clinical appearance even in the absence of fungous infection elsewhere on the skin, but should always be confirmed microscopically by finding hyphae in the nail plate. The easiest way to find the fungus is to soak full thickness clippings from the diseased nails in a very small quantity of 5% potassium hydroxide for 24 hours. The nail is quite soft at the end of this time and the filaments are readily seen under the microscope using the $\frac{2}{3}$ inch objective and reduced light and confirming with the $\frac{1}{6}$ inch. No staining is required. A single negative should not be accepted if the clinical appearances support the diagnosis. It is not essential to prepare

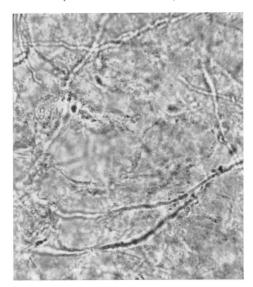

Fig. 38 Trichophyton filaments in potash preparation. Reduced by 50% from ×962

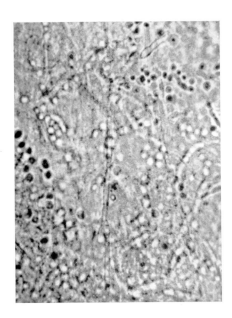

Fig. 39 Candida albicans infection of nail plate—potash preparation. (Pseudohyphae and groups of yeasts.) Reduced by 30% from ×612

cultures in every case but it is advisable to do so whenever possible. A negative culture is not uncommon in the presence of abundant mycelium seen in potash preparations; mixed infections are encountered occasionally. The appearances of mycelia

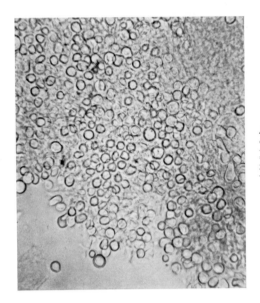

Fig. 40 Scopulariopsis brevicaulis infection of nail plate—potash preparation (group of large spores some pear shaped). Reduced by 50% from ×962

seen in potash preparations are shown in Fig. 38 and compared with candida (Fig. 39) and scopulariopsis (Fig. 40). The appearances are sufficiently different for the diagnosis to be established with some confidence before the result of culture is available.

Treatment

The treatment of finger nail infections has been greatly improved since griseofulvin became available. Local applications of any kind have little or no influence on fungous infections of the nail. The organisms penetrate the nail so deeply that no application so far available will penetrate sufficiently to carry a fungicide deep enough to eradicate the infection. The portion of nailplate covered by the dorsal nail fold is often infected and it is impossible to reach this area by local applications.

Before treatment with griseofulvin is started the presence of fungus must be confirmed. In the majority of finger nail infections clinical cure may be obtained. Failure is probably due to inadequate absorption of the drug or too small a dose. In the early stages of treatment a rather large dose is recommended. For adults weighing 70 kg and over 1 g a day of the fine particle preparation should be given for the first two weeks, reducing then to 750 mg for 2 to 4 weeks. Subsequently the patient should take 500 mg daily until clinical cure is obtained. This is usually between 5 and 6 months from the start of treatment and depends on the rate of growth of the nail. Either the 125 mg tablets or the 500 mg tablet may be used but the smaller tablets are preferred by the author. For smaller adults the initial dose should be 750 mg daily reducing to 500 mg and for children 500 mg reducing to 375 or 250 mg. The large doses at the start of treatment may cause minor side effects such as headaches and gastric discomfort but the patient should be encouraged to take the full dose. It is occasionally necessary to abandon treatment because of more serious side effects.

The treatment of toe nail infections is much less satisfactory. If the finger nails are not involved it is usually better not to attempt treatment. If, however, one is dealing with a young patient and only a few toe nails are infected, these may be removed surgically and treatment with griseofulvin started at the same time. The first few mm of nail to emerge from under the nail fold may still be infected and should be cut or filed away as soon as possible. Treatment with griseofulvin should be continued for about 6 months as with finger nails. The author has had occasional success using griseofulvin only.

If toe nails are heavily infected and treatment for the finger nails is instituted considerable improvement may be noted in the toe nails and at times it is justifiable to continue the griseofulvin for 12 to 18 months, if it seems probable that clinically normal toe nails will be obtained. There is however a danger of producing ingrowing toe nails in some cases as the normal nail is a good deal wider than the previously diseased nail; the surrounding soft tissue has shrunk over the years so that there is now insufficient space for the full sized nail. Treatment must then be given to relieve the discomfort and may require total removal of the nail.

Occasionally the fungal infection appears to be replaced by a candidal infection and this may account for some apparent failures in treatment with griseofulvin.

Relapse after clinical cure is unfortunately not very uncommon. Fungus may often be found microscopically after the nails appear normal clinically, so that relapse may be due to reactivation of fungus previously quiescent, or to re-infection. Treatment following relapse is generally less satisfactory than on the first occasion griseofulvin is used.

Scopulariopsis Brevicaulis

This is a fungus found widely in nature which is occasionally found in nails. The infection is almost always confined to one or both great toe nails and produces a yellow or chalky discoloration of part of the nail (Plate I (d)). It seems probable that the

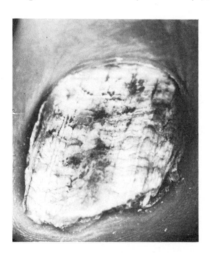

Fig. 41 Nail infected with aspergillus candidus

organism invades and lives on the keratin of a nail which has been damaged previously in some way. The irregular appearance of the mycelium and the groups of large spores in potash preparations often give a clue to the diagnosis, but it should be confirmed by culture.

The condition is persistent and is usually best left untreated because it may recur even after surgical removal of the nail.

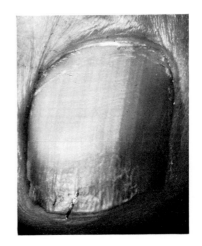

Fig. 42   Same nail as in *Fig. 41*, two months later

Other non-dermatophytes e.g. Aspergillus species are found occasionally. They too can probably invade only a previously damaged nail. One case of Aspergillus candidus treated by the author cleared very quickly under treatment with topical applications of miconazole acetate only (Figs. 41 and 42).

References

Hildrick-Smith, G, Blank, H and Sarkany, I (1964). Fungus diseases and their treatment. Little Brown & Co., Boston

Davies, R R, Everall, J D and Hamilton, E (1967) Mycological and clinical evaluation of griseofulvin for chronic onychomycosis. *Brit. med. J.* **2** 464

Martin-Scott, I (1954) Onychomycosis caused by Scopulariopsis brevicaulis. *Trans. Brit. Mycol. Soc.* **37** 38

Riddell, R W (1965). Fungous diseases of Britain. *Brit. med. J.* **2** 783

Walshe, M M and English, M P (1966) Fungi in nails. *Brit. J. Derm.* **78** 198

Chapter 5

Chronic Paronychia

Chronic paronychia is very common. It is the commonest nail complaint to take the patient to the doctor. Psoriasis and fungal infections probably have a greater overall incidence but are usually only part of more widespread disease. It is encountered in persons who have their hands very often exposed to moisture and is therefore common among housewives, bartenders, laundry workers and in many other trades. In temperate climates it is more common in persons with cold hands. The great majority of cases occur in women. It may occur at any age but most are between 30 and 60 at the time of onset (Esteves, 1959). Affected men are usually in one of the trades of chef, barman or fishmonger (Frain-Bell, 1957). It is occasionally seen in young children especially as a result of thumb-sucking (Stone and Mullins, 1968). It is common in diabetics (Hellier, 1955). Any finger may be affected but those most often involved are the index and middle fingers of the right hand and the middle finger of the left (Frain-Bell, 1957). These are the fingers most subject to minor trauma.

There is considerable dispute as to the aetiological factors involved in the causation of chronic paronychia. It seldom follows acute infections although acute exacerbations occur from time to time.

In most cases the initial change is a loss of the cuticle from the whole or part of the nail. This normally results from maceration in water especially if alkaline, but occasionally is the result of manicure or other trauma. The loss of the cuticle allows the space between the posterior nail fold and the nail plate to open (Fig. 43) and this area becomes colonised by candida species, usually Candida albicans. Barlow et al. (1970) believe that Staphylococcus pyogenes plays an active role in the early stages

50

helping to penetrate the keratin at the base of the nail and in opening up the nail fold. When well established candida can be found in almost every case if a bead of pus is present or if the keratin of the under surface of the posterior nail fold is gently scraped. Acute exacerbations causing considerable discomfort are probably the result of secondary bacterial infection and

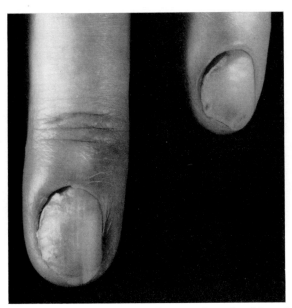

Fig. 43 Chronic paronychia early stage. Loss of cuticle and bolstering of posterior nail fold

subside fairly quickly. Various bacteria may be involved including staphylococci, streptococci, Escherichia coli and Pseudomonas aeruginosa. To what extent the candidal infection is responsible for the perpetuation of the condition is at present uncertain but many believe it is of paramount importance. Stone and Mullins (1965) have shown that the process can be initiated by introducing non-viable Candida albicans into a relatively sterile nail fold. Foreign material passes through the epidermis of the roof of the nail fold and acting as a foreign body sets up a chronic inflammation in the adjacent dermis. This foreign material may well be derived from the candida. The reaction in the dermis produces the rounding off of the dorsal nail fold and the bolstering which is so characteristic of the established case. Once the foreign material has penetrated to the dermis it is very difficult to remove.

Clinical appearances

One or many nails may be involved. There is redness and bolstering of the dorsal nail fold (Fig. 43) with some discomfort.

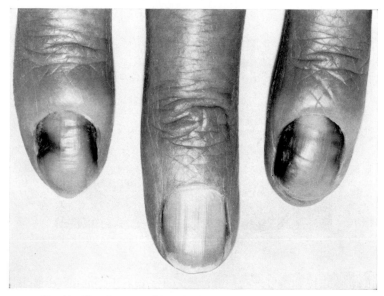

Fig. 44 Chronic paronychia—discoloration of edges of affected nails

Often a small bead of pus may be expressed from one corner of the nail fold. From time to time there is more intense inflammation with increase of pain. The nail plate itself, in the early stages is unaffected but soon the edge becomes irregular and discoloured brown or black (Fig. 44) and this may extend over a considerable portion of the nail. The nail plate may become cross ridged (Fig. 45). After a time the size of the nail is liable to become considerably reduced and this appearance is exaggerated

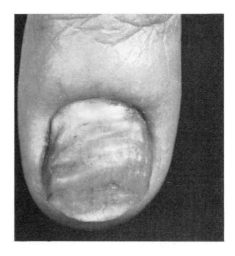

Fig. 45 Chronic paronychia—
cross ridging of nail plate

by the swelling and induration of the surrounding soft tissues (Figs. 46 and 47). Occasionally the whole nail plate takes on a

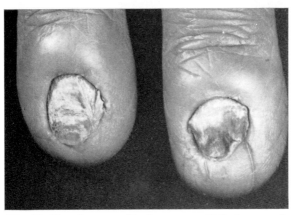

Fig. 46 Chronic paronychia late stage. Nail plates much
involved and size of nail reduced

brownish discoloration similar to tinea unguium but the bolstering at the nail base may persist and aid in differentiation. In

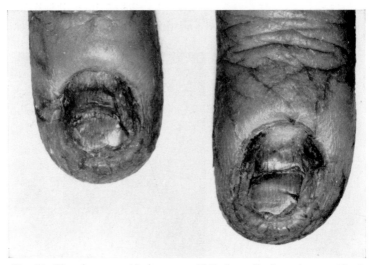

Fig. 47 Chronic paronychia late stage. Nail plates discoloured, cross ridged and reduced in size

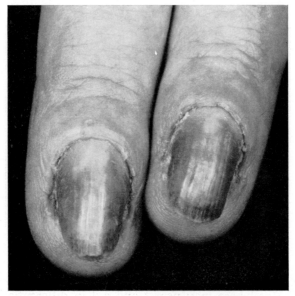

Fig. 48 Candida albicans infection of nail plates

PLATE III

[a] Leukonychia totalis

[b] Pseudomonas
aeruginosa infection

[c] Radiodermatitis

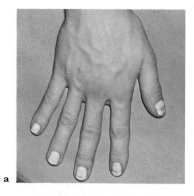

a

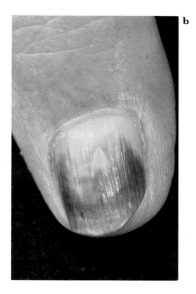

b

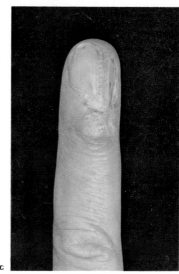

c

[d] Onycholysis
and subungual
haemorrhage
due to dilute
hydrofluoric acid

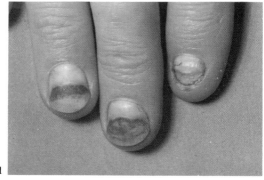

d

PLATE IV

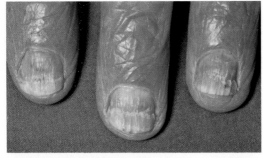

[a] Raynaud's phenomenon —nail changes

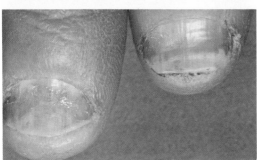

[b] Raynaud's phenomenon —nail changes

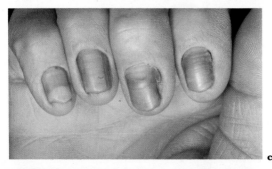

[c] The nails in the 'yellow nail' syndrome

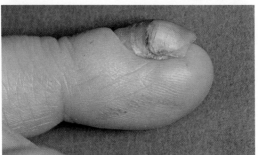

[d] The nails in the 'yellow nail' syndrome

these cases it will be found that Candida has invaded the nail plate (Fig. 48 and Plate I (*c*)). Most of the deformity of the nail is however the result of inflammation in the region of the matrix interfering with the growth of the nail but there is some evidence that the discoloration at the edge of the nail is due to bacteria, especially Pseudomonas aeruginosa invading the nail (Stone and Mullins, 1963).

The condition is an extremely persistent one and without treatment may last for years. It often remains confined to one or two fingers but several fingers may be involved. In such cases some will resolve spontaneously after a few weeks or months whilst others remain infected.

Treatment

As with any chronic disorder where there is no specific remedy many forms of treatment have been recommended for chronic paronychia. No single remedy will work in every case. Certain general principles are important. The patient must be instructed to keep her hands as dry as possible. This is perhaps the most important part of treatment and the one which proves to be the most difficult to carry out in some cases. If further maceration cannot be prevented no local application will produce a cure. In patients who suffer from cold hands a peripheral vasodilator should be prescribed in adequate dosage.

In the early stages when there is erythema and discomfort a short course of an antibiotic directed against the staphylococcus may be helpful. As the organism is usually insensitive to penicillin and the tetracyclines, erythromycin is the drug of choice (Barlow *et al.*, 1970).

For local application many things can be used. As the condition is likely to last for weeks or months a colourless preparation is preferred by most patients. Nystatin (mycostatin) ointment or cream works very well in some cases and is usually worth a trial. Alternatively amphoteracin B as a lotion, cream or ointment may be tried although the yellow staining may be an embarrassment. These two preparations combat the candidal element but do not deal with the gram negative organisms. Clotrimazole (Canesten cream or solution) and miconazole (Daktarin; Demonistat) are two other useful preparations which may be tried. The author has found 15% sulphacetamide in 50% spirit (alcohol) very useful especially in long standing cases. This is both anticandidal and antibacterial. The medicaments are applied to the dorsal nail fold 3 or 4 times a day, a brush is needed to apply the liquids.

When coloured preparations are tolerated 1% gentian violet in 25% spirit or Castellani's paint may be tried. Whatever treatment is selected it must be continued for weeks or months and the patient cannot be considered cured until all swelling has subsided and the cuticle restored. In some cases complete cure is never obtained. Dr Stahle (personal communication) finds that small injections of triamcinolone into the dorsal nail fold, although painful, are often of great value in reducing the swelling and overcoming the inflammation.

Only very rarely is it advisable to remove the nail plate e.g. in the presence of severe acute exacerbation and if this is done great care must be taken during regrowth of the nail or the end result will be no better than before treatment was started. An antiseptic paint or cream should be used and the area protected from further maceration.

When there is obvious candidal infection elsewhere this should also be treated.

Infections of the Nail Plate with Candida Albicans

In many cases of chronic paronychia, Candida albicans can be recovered from the edge of the nail of infected fingers but this does not represent true invasion of the nail with the organism. However true invasion can occur at times and it is usually a complication of chronic paronychia or of long standing onycholysis. Occasionally no history of preceeding paronychia or onycholysis can be obtained and in these cases the condition will mimic tinea unguium very closely. It may not be possible to differentiate with certainty without culture of the organism although this can often be done on the appearances in the potash preparations (p. 46). Candidal infection of finger nails appears to be becoming more common but infection of toe nails remains very uncommon. Species other than C albicans e.g. C krusei, C parapsilosis and C tropicalis are encountered occasionally.

There are two rather characteristic clinical appearances to candidal infection of the nail plates when several nails are involved. The first is illustrated well in Fig. 48. The nails remain fairly smooth but they are overcurved in their long axis, are discoloured brown and become opaque. The second type is illustrated in Plate I (c). In this form the nails are flat and often show extensive onycholysis. The nail itself is rough and irregular and is again discoloured brown. The nail bed may be thickened. In this type the local circulation is usually very poor.

Candida albicans is unaffected by griseofulvin so that treatment is very difficult and if simple measures fail it may be necessary to remove the infected nails. If onycholysis is present the nail bed may become thick and rough, and in these cases the bed should be curetted at the same time as the nail is removed. Cure cannot be guaranteed and this radical procedure should only be undertaken as a last resort.

There are a few conditions in which invasion of the nail by Candida albicans is an important feature. One of these is acrodermatitis enteropathica, a rare developmental anomaly seen in young children. Another is a genetically determined form of muco-cutaneous candidiasis. In this condition there appears to be a failure to metabolise iron and the administration of iron parenterally may result in the nail infection being overcome (Higgs and Wells, 1972).

References

Barlow, A J E, Chattaway, F W, Holgate, M C and Aldersley, T (1970) Chronic paronychia. *Brit. J. Derm.* **82** 448

Esteves, J (1959) Pathogenesis and treatment of chronic paronychia. *Dermatologica* **119** 229

Frain-Bell, W (1957). Chronic paronychia. Short review of 590 cases. Trans. *St. John's Hosp. Derm. Soc. (Lond.)* **38** 29

Hellier, F F (1965) Chronic paronychia. *Brit. med. J.* **2** 1358

Higgs, J M and Wells, R S (1972) Chronic muco-cutaneous candidiasis: associated abnormalities of iron metabolism *Brit. J. Derm.* **86** *Supp.* 8 88

Stone, O J and Mullins, J F (1963) Role of Pseudomonas aeruginosa in nail disease. *J. invest. Derm.* **41** 25

Stone, O J and Mullins, J F (1965) Role of Candida albicans in chronic disease. *Arch. Derm.* **91** 70

Stone, O J and Mullins, J F (1968) Chronic paronychia in children. *Clin. Pediat. (Phila.)* **7** 104

Chapter 6

Nail Disorders Associated with other Dermatological Conditions

Dermatitis

Dermatitis can play havoc with the nails and in most cases the cause of the nail damage is obvious. At times however the dermatitis is under control before the patient complains of the nail changes and in these one has to rely on the history for confirmatory diagnosis. Such patients are usually referred as suspected fungous infection of the nails; this is generally easily excluded.

Nail changes may occur in any type of dermatitis involving the hands and in particular the skin adjacent to the nail, but atopic dermatitis more frequently affects the nails than do other types. In atopic dermatitis and in pompholyx the nail changes sometimes predominate. One must assume in these cases that the eczematous process is most marked on the under surface of the dorsal nail fold.

The usual change is an atrophic process and consists of the development of irregular ridges across the nail (Figs. 49 and 50). In addition coarse pitting may affect one or more nails (Figs. 49 and 51). The ridges occur independently on one or several nails and the overall change is a very ugly nail. If the ridges go deep enough they may lead to temporary shedding of part of the nail (Fig. 50). In the early stages only the proximal part of the nails will be involved (Fig. 52). Subungual haemorrhages either petechial or more extensive may complicate the picture, as may chronic paronychia. The ridges must be distinguished from ridges formed by other causes and in particular the traumatic nail dystrophy produced by a habit tic (p. 133).

The sudden onset of generalised dermatitis may be accompanied by the formation of a depression on all nails similar to

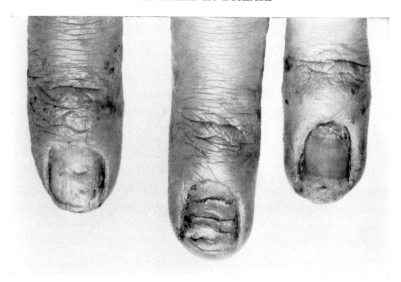

Fig. 49 Dermatitis—coarse pitting and cross ridging

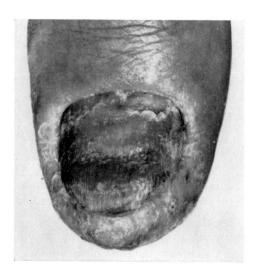

Fig. 50 Dermatitis—cross ridging and partial loss of nail plate

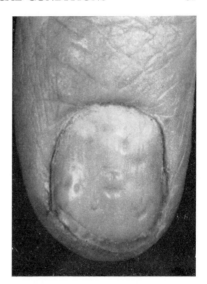

Fig. 51 Dermatitis—coarse pitting
only

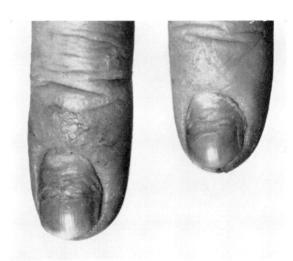

Fig. 52 Dermatitis—commencement of nail deformities

Beau's lines (p. 112) but in dermatitis the nail behind the depression is likely to be deformed (Fig. 53). In exfoliative dermatitis the nails may be shed.

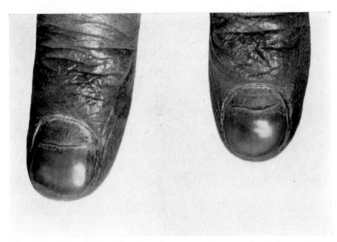

Fig. 53　The nails following the onset of generalised dermatitis—depression on all nails followed by a deformed nail

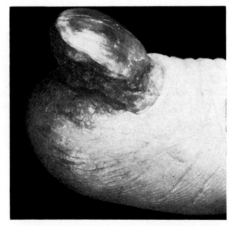

Fig. 54　Dermatitis—hypertrophied nails

Although the usual nail change in dermatitis is an atrophic process occasionally gross hypertrophy occurs. These cases are associated with inflammation of the nail fold, and the nail becomes very thick and irregular (Fig. 54). This type of hypertrophy is probably always due to exogenous causes. It must be distinguished from psoriasis precipitated by trauma or chemical irritation. In these cases there will be no evidence of dermatitis

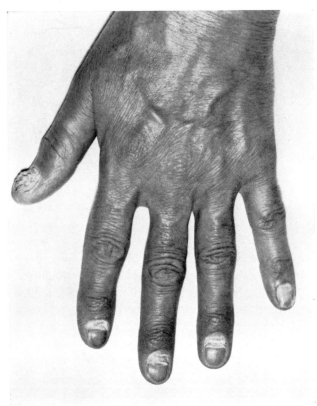

Fig. 55 Psoriasis precipitated by chemical trauma and simulating dermatitis of the nails

of the fingers but there may also be no other evidence of psoriasis (Fig. 55).

Benedek (1946) believes that the nail changes in pompholyx, seborrhoeic dermatitis and psoriasis are all due to the same cause and are the result of the activities of an organism which he calls Bacillus endoparasiticus (Benedek, 1927). He says that the changes are usually called onychomycosis but that that condition is really very rare. It is true that dermatitis of the nails is often mistaken for onychomycosis but it can readily be differentiated by the absence of fungal mycelia in nail clippings. When fungi are present onychomycosis can be diagnosed with certainty and the result of treatment with griseofulvin confirms this finding. Psoriasis can usually be differentiated on clinical grounds. The Bacillus endoparasiticus is probably Pityrosporum ovale and can play little or no part in nail pathology.

Onycholysis is not infrequently seen in association with dermatitis of the finger tips presumably as a result of irritant material being trapped under the free edge of the nail and then penetrating further backwards. Occasionally the irritant material may pass through the nail plate to reach the nail bed. Shelley (1972) has noted onycholysis from the topical application of 5% 5 fluorouracil to the finger tips under occlusion. The condition was reversible and was not produced by a 2% preparation.

Highly polished nails are sometimes seen in patients with generalised erythroderma. This is, of course, an indirect effect as the patients rub their hands on their skin to obtain relief from itching, preferring this to actual scratching as it does less damage. Another change sometimes encountered is the so called 'usure des ongles' a wearing away of the nails due to scratching.

Treatment is essentially treatment of the dermatitis. The nails will return to normal gradually but complete restoration cannot be expected in less than three months. If chronic paronychia complicates the dermatitis it must be treated independently.

Lichen striatus

This is essentially an eczematous process in which the changes are restricted to a linear band often transversing the whole length of a limb. If it extends as far as the distal phalanx it may cause changes in the nail of the affected digit similar to the changes seen in dermatitis. It is usually restricted to a single finger. The author has seen a number of these cases but there are very few recorded in the literature. Kaufman (1974) records one such case.

Lichen Planus

The author (Samman, 1961) has shown that some nail changes occur in about 10% of cases of lichen planus but that the damage is usually mild and transient. Permanent loss with scarring may

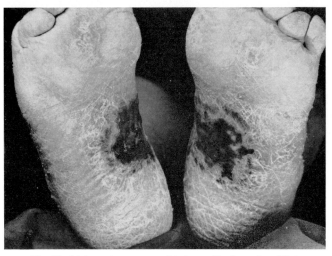

Fig. 56 Lichen planus—atrophic type affecting soles of feet

however occur and is the most serious injury. Any nail may be involved but most often it is the great toe nail. There is a rare variety of lichen planus which produces an atrophic process on the sole and permanent destruction of many toe nails (Figs. 56 and 57). There may be very little evidence of lichen planus on other parts of the body (Cram *et al.*, 1966; Degos and Schnitzler, 1967). The commonest change seen on the nails in lichen planus is an increase in the longitudinal striations of the nail plate. The ridges may be accompanied by slight depressions on the surface

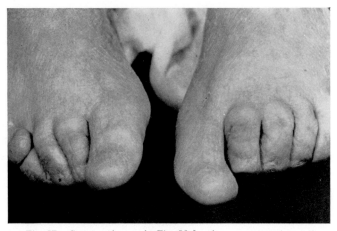

Fig. 57 Same patient as in *Fig. 56* showing accompanying nail destruction

which catch the light (Fig. 58). Ridging usually occurs in severe generalised lichen planus and may be seen starting near the cuticle and moving forward with the growth of the nail. The nail

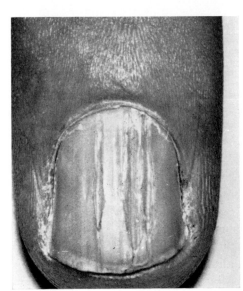

Fig. 58 Lichen planus—ridging and slight depressions on nail surface

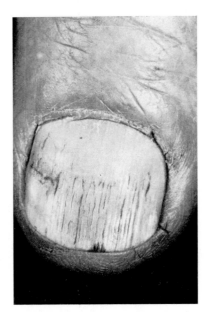

Fig. 59   Lichen planus—ridging. Nail returning to normal

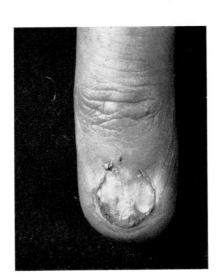

Fig. 60 Lichen planus—nail thinning and pterygium formation

plate is often slightly thinned but after a time returns to normal
(Fig. 59). If the nail thinning is more severe the cuticle may grow
forward over the base of the nail and attach itself to the nail plate
(Fig. 60). An exaggeration of this process leads to pterygium
formation and may progress to permanent loss of a part or whole
of the nail. Permanent loss however is not necessarily preceded
by pterygium formation. Temporary shedding of one or more

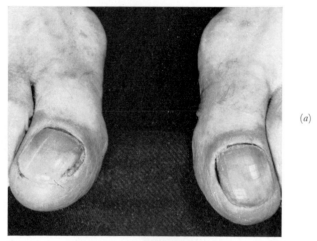

(a)

Fig. 61 (*a*) (*b*) and (*c*)   Lichen planus—shedding of nails
followed by partial replacement

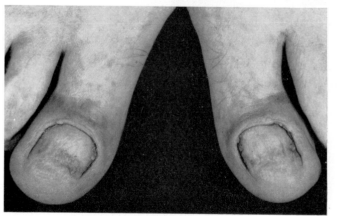

(b)

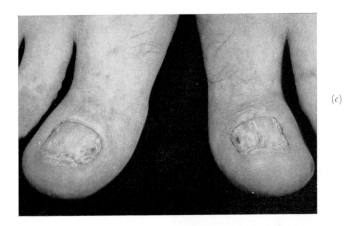

(c)

nails is also encountered at times and the new nail when it forms
may be incomplete (Fig. 61).

It can be shown histologically that the damage to the nail is
the result of lichen planus in the region of the matrix and when
scarring occurs it is analogous to the scarring seen following
lichen planus around the hair roots. Zaias (1970) has shown that
pterygium formation is due to an adhesion forming between
the epidermis of the dorsal nail fold and the nail bed. He also
says that lichen planus of the nail bed may give rise to hyperpigmentation, subungual hyperkeratosis and onycholoysis.

Lichen planus of the nails without evidence of lichen planus
elsewhere undoubtedly occurs (Burgoon and Kostrazewa, 1969;
Cornelius and Shelley, 1967) and has been seen by the author on
a number of occasions. Lichen planus in childhood is uncommon
but several examples of nail destruction in children due to lichen
planus have been seen by the author (Marks and Samman, 1972).

If it is possible to make a confident diagnosis of lichen planus
whilst severe nail changes are taking place, treatment with
systemic corticosteriods may be justified in an attempt to save
the nails. The possible harmful effects must be balanced against
the chance of saving the nails and in this context it should be
realised that permanent damage can occur quite quickly.

Darier's Disease

In this rare genetically determined disorder the nails are affected in a high percentage of cases. There have been a number of good descriptive papers (Ronchese, 1965; Schubert, 1966;

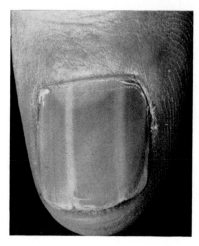

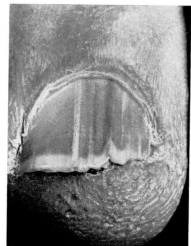

Fig. 62 Darier's disease—characteristic white streaks

Fig. 63 Darier's disease—dark streak and ridging with notch at free margin

Savin and Samman, 1970). The nails may show a variety of changes. The most characteristic is the presence of a white streak or streaks (Fig. 62) extending longitudinally through the nail and crossing the half moon. One or more nails may be affected. Later the streaks lose their white colour and become darker and ridges may appear on the nails which then tend to crack (Fig. 63). Where a streak meets the free edge of the nail a V-shaped notch may appear (Fig. 63). Much less often the nail becomes greatly thickened (Fig. 64). Ronchese (1965) suggests that at times nail changes may occur in the absence of other evidence of the disease. This is one of the few occasions when a biopsy may be helpful as characteristic changes may be found in the nail folds and nail matrix (Zaias and Ackerman, 1973).

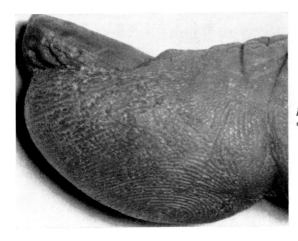

Fig. 64 Darier's disease—gross thickening

Alopecia Areata

Shedding of the nails in alopecia areata is very uncommon. Some alteration of the nail plate is however quite frequent and in cases observed by the author about 10% have shown some change. Rubisz Brzezimksa and Seferowicz say they found pits in 62% of 100 patients and other trophic changes in 4%. The common abnormality is pitting and the most characteristic is a uniform pitting affecting several nails (Fig. 65). The pits are small as in psoriasis and when uniform make lines of pits both across and in the long axis of the nail. If the pits are produced very rapidly greater distortion of the nail plate occurs, the nail loses its lustre and becomes roughened (Fig. 66). In nails with an exposed half moon there may be a meshwork of a pale yellow

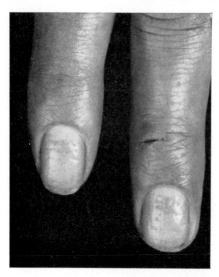

Fig. 65   Alopecia areata—uniform pitting

Fig. 66 Alopecia areata—pitting and distortion of nail plate

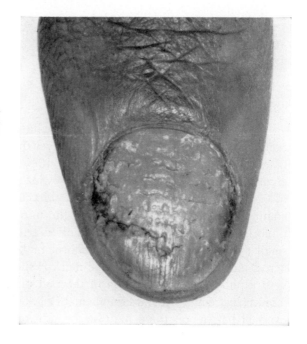

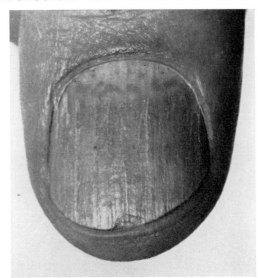

Fig. 67 Alopecia areata (universalis) showing mottling in half-moon area

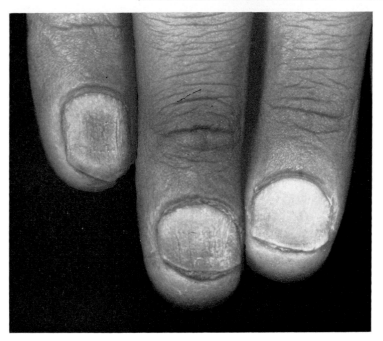

Fig. 68 Alopecia areata, severe finger nail changes

colour visible through the nail plate in this area (Fig. 67) as seen also in psoriasis (p. 25).

Much grosser changes are seen occasionally. Most nails (finger and toe) are involved. They become rough, opalescent, some are thinned and some are thickened (Figs. 68 and 69). Several will show koilonychia. The changes are identical with those described under the heading of 'severe nail dystrophy' (p. 184).

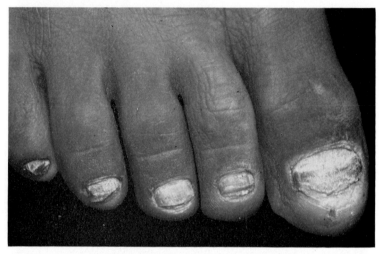

Fig. 69   Alopecia areata, severe toe nail damage

Nail changes are most often seen in association with severe alopecia (Fig. 70) but not always so and occasionally the nail changes predominate. The changes may be observed to appear following the onset of alopecia but once established may persist after the hair fall has ceased. The author has seen patients referred on account of their nail dystrophy who have developed alopecia areata months later. Some cases of nail pitting without alopecia must have the same aetiology. Treatment has little effect on the process.

Two cases associated with total vitiligo were described by Demis and Weiner (1963).

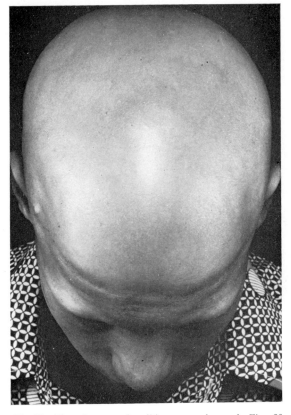

Fig. 70 Alopecia areata (totalis), same patient as in *Figs. 68*
and *69*

Pityriasis Rubra Pilaris

In this disease the nail changes may closely simulate the grosser changes of psoriasis with thickening of the nail plate and the nail bed (Fig. 71). On other occasions cross ridging may occur as in dermatitis.

Reiter's Syndrome

When the skin is involved in this condition the lesions are scaly or crusted and described as keratoderma. When this occurs,

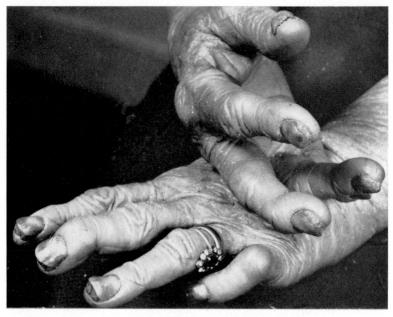

Fig. 71 Pityriasis rubra pilaris

and it is rather rare, the nails are likely to be involved and then show changes which are similar to the grosser changes of psoriasis. The nails may also be displaced by the development of hyperkeratosis of the nail bed (Fig. 72). Deep pits or even punched-out areas are seen occasionally (Fig. 73).

Scleroderma

In scleroderma of the progressive type (acrosclerosis) the nails may remain remarkably normal even in the presence of severe Raynaud's symptoms and atrophy of the pulp of the distal phalanx (Fig. 5). However any of the nails may become defective with the changes corresponding to those described under impaired peripheral circulation (Chapter 8). Not infrequently isolated nails are partly or wholly destroyed (Fig. 101). A rather characteristic change is described as "beaking" when the nails look like a parrot's beak curving around the atrophic soft tissue of the finger

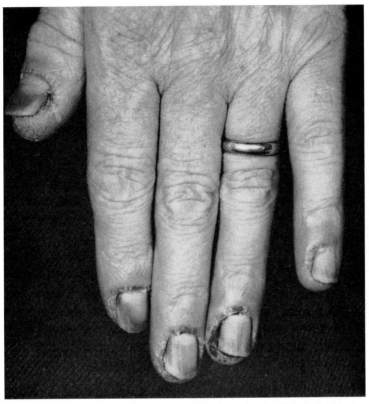

Fig. 72 Reiter's syndrome—hyperkeratosis around and under nail

Fig. 73 Reiter's syndrome—
punched out area of nail plate

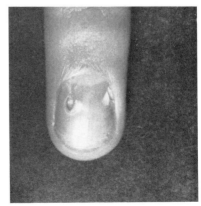

tip. This is well shown in the left thumb in Fig. 5 (p. 8), but the change can be more exaggerated than shown there.

Disseminate Lupus Erythematosus and Dermatomyositis

Although the nail plates themselves are unlikely to be affected in these conditions, changes in the skin close to the nail may be of great help in diagnosis. In each condition there may be patches of erythema with telangiectasia over the posterior nail folds. In disseminate lupus erythematosus the cuticles may be broken and there may be haemorrhagic lesions in the area. In dermatomyositis linear bands of erythema may occur over the knuckles in addition to the erythema at the base of the nail.

Radiodermatitis

Many years after an excessive dose of X-ray locally, either therapeutic or accidental (e.g. in dental surgeons and radiologists), the nails may become rough and discoloured. The telltale telangiectasia and atrophy of the surrounding soft tissues leave no doubt about the diagnosis (Plate III (c)). The excess X-ray may result from a single application e.g. for treatment of a periungual wart (Fig. 74) or more often from repeated small doses over a period of months or years.

Pemphigus

Various dystrophic changes may occur if bullae of pemphigus vulgaris involve the finger tips. In pemphigus foliaceus cross ridging may occur and shedding of the nails has been reported.

Epidermolysis Bullosa Dystrophica

There are several varieties of this rare disorder. Permanent loss (Fig. 75) of one or more nails is comparatively common and occurs before the patients reach adult life. It is usually impossible to say at what age the nail was actually lost but blistering in the

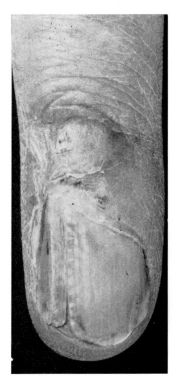

Fig. 74 Radiodermatitis following treatment of a periungual wart

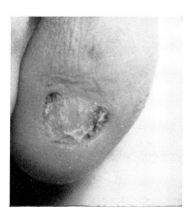

Fig. 75 Epidermolysis bullosa

neighbourhood of the nail probably precedes the scarring. On other occasions the affected nails may be only partly destroyed.

Acanthosis Nigricans

In this rare disease the nails may become thickened and discoloured (Fig. 76).

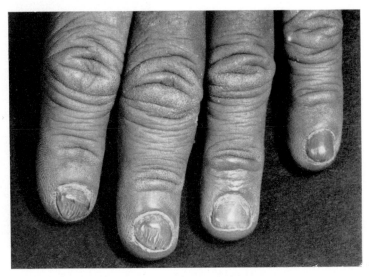

Fig. 76   Acanthosis nigricans

Sarcoidosis

Sarcoidosis of the lupus pernio type often affects the digits of fingers or toes. If the damage is situated close to the nail, the latter may be deformed in various ways. It may become thickened and very irregular (Fig. 78), it may become defective especially near the tip (Fig. 77), or it may be lost altogether. X-ray will often show that the underlying bone has been damaged (Fig. 79).

Norwegian Scabies

This rare variety of scabies is seen mainly in mentally defective persons. The patient suffers little discomfort from irritation

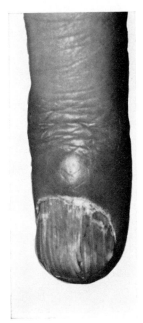

Fig. 77   Sarcoidosis

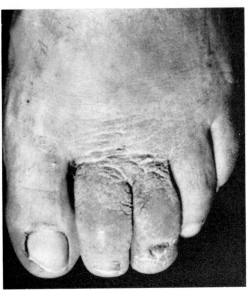

Fig. 78   Sarcoidosis interfering
with nail formation

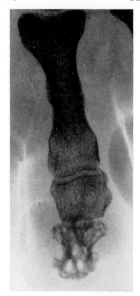

Fig. 79 X-ray of middle toe of foot seen in *Fig. 78* showing sarcoidosis in distal phalanx

Fig. 80 Norwegian (or crusted) scabies

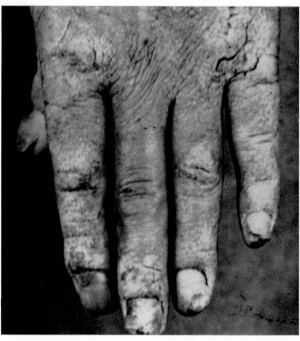

although he may harbour many thousands of acari. The nails may be greatly distorted becoming thick and opaque (Figs. 80 and 81) and on microscopic examination will be found to contain countless acari and their eggs. The diagnosis is often missed

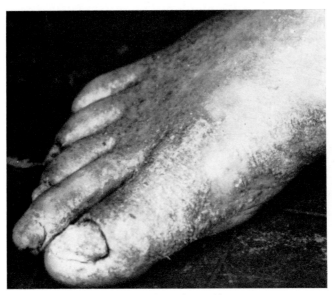

Fig. 81 Norwegian scabies

until contact cases develop signs of ordinary scabies. Treatment with benzyl benzoate is effective.

Syphilis

The nails may be involved in primary syphilis or in the later stages of the disease. Primary syphilis may resemble a whitlow. Various dystrophic changes may occur in late syphilis but are now very rarely seen in the UK.

Leprosy

In leprosy the nails may become dystrophic or actually destroyed as a result of anaesthesia when it affects the extremities.

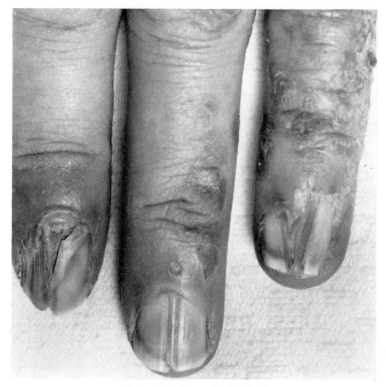

Fig. 82   Porokeratosis of Mibelli

Porokeratosis (Mibelli)

The nails are occasionally damaged in this rare disorder. Figure 82 shows splitting, ridging and partial destruction of 3 nails, changes which closely resemble those of impaired peripheral circulation.

References

Benedek, T (1946) Pompholyx. *Urological and Cutaneous Review* **50** 467

Burgoon, C F Jr. and Kostrazewa, R M (1969) Lichen Planus limited to the nails. *Arch. Derm.* **100** 371

Cornelius, C E III and Shelley, W B (1967) Permanent Anonychia due to Lichen Planus. *Arch. Derm.* **96** 434

Cram, D L, Kierland, R R and Winkelmann, R K (1966) Ulcerative Lichen Planus of the Feet. *Arch. Derm.* **93** 692

Degos, R and Schnitzler, L (1967) Lichen erosive des Orteils. *Ann. Derm. Syph.* (Paris) **94** 241

Demis, D J and Weiner, M R (1963) Alopecia Universalis, Onychodystrophy and Total Vitiligo. *Arch. Derm.* **88** 195

Kaufman, J P (1974) Lichen striatus with nail involvement. *Cutis* **14** 232

Marks, R and Samman, P D (1972) Isolated Nail Dystrophy due to Lichen Planus, *Trans. St. John's Hosp. Derm. Soc.* **58** 93

Ronchese, F (1965) The Nail in Darier's Disease. *Arch. Derm.* **91** 617

Rubisz Brzerzinska, J and Seferowicz, E (1974) Studies on the incidence of lesions in the nail plates in alopecia areata (Polish) *Przegel Derm.* **61** 147

Savin, J A and Samman P D (1970) The Nail in Darier's Disease. *Medical and Biological Illustration* **20** 85

Schubert, H (1966) Nagelveranderungen bei Morbus Darier. *Zeits für Haut-und Gesch.* **41** 239

Shelley, W B (1972) Onycholysis due to topical 5 fluorouracil. *Acta. Derm. Vererol Stock.* **52** 320

Zaias, N (1970) The Nail in Lichen Planus. *Arch. Derm.* **101** 264

Zaias, N and Ackerman, A B (1975) The Nail in Darier-White disease. *Arch. Derm.* **107** 193

Chapter 7

Miscellaneous Acquired Nail Disorders

Bacterial Paronychia

This is an extremely common condition but rather infrequently seen by the dermatologist. It is an acute process due to infection with Staph. pyogenes in most instances and is often the result of minor trauma, especially injury by a foreign body such as a splinter, or injury inflicted by nail biting. Infection with other organisms may occur, including Strep. pyogenes, and Pseudomonas aeruginosa; the latter is especially common in an acute exacerbation of chronic paronychia. In addition to infections round the nail, infections may occur under the nail plate when the nail may be loosened or actually shed.

Bacterial paronychia is a painful condition and the pain persists until the pus is freed or until the infection comes under control with antibiotics. Granulation tissue may develop in the nail folds (Fig. 83). Very superficial infections often point somewhere along the nail fold and treatment is readily effected by pricking with a sterile needle or sharp pointed scalpel. For deeper infections antibiotic treatment is usually necessary. It is unlikely that a sample of pus can be obtained for sensitivity tests of the organism, so that treatment must be empirical and a broad spectrum antibiotic is preferred. If the condition does not quickly subside, surgical drainage will be required. When infection is under the nail plate and especially if the nail plate has been loosened, removal of the nail is advised.

Herpetic Whitlow

This also is seldom seen by the dermatologist but Stern *et al.* (1959) have shown that infection of the finger tips with the herpes simplex virus is common in hospital nurses and orderlies as a form of cross infection. The condition closely mimics bacterial

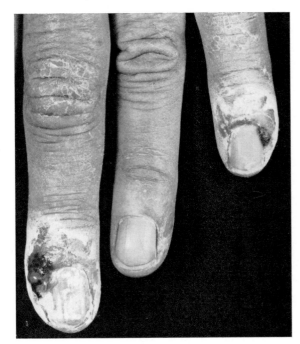

Fig. 83 Acute par-
onychia

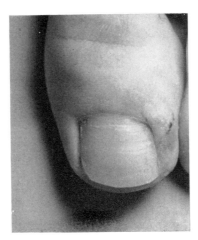

Fig. 84 Herpetic whitlow

infection but is more resistant to treatment and there is never true pus formation. Eight cases are described by La Rossa and Hamilton (1971), 5 of these were in medical or dental personnel. Their paper is well illustrated in colour. The condition may affect one or more fingers and starts with a single vesicle but others may develop soon afterwards. Herpetic whitlows may also occur on the toes (Fig. 84). The diagnosis may be confirmed by cytology of the blister fluid or by recovering the virus. There may be secondary bacterial contamination.

The condition is painful and the pain usually lasts about ten days. It takes about three weeks for the lesions to dry up entirely and occasionally the nail is shed temporarily. It may be accompanied by lymphangitis. Treatment is palliative, dilute potassium permanganate soaks and a dry dressing are recommended. Idoxyuridine 5% in dimethylsulphoxide may be used in severe cases to shorten an attack.

Onycholysis
(idiopathic)

Onycholysis as a symptom is mentioned on p. 20. There are many known causes but when they have been excluded many cases remain where no cause can be found.

Spontaneous onycholysis is common and can be very troublesome. The loosened nail is unsightly and dirt which collects beneath it is difficult to remove. In the early stages the condition is painless but the nail loses its value as an aid in the picking up of small objects. The condition is almost confined to women and is seen especially in persons who like to keep their nails long so that minor trauma may play a part in aetiology. Patients often notice that the affected nails grow faster than their normal nails and measurements have confirmed this (Dawber et al., 1971). The reason for the increased growth rate is not yet known.

One or several nails may be involved and usually only part of the nail is separated (Fig. 85), but once loosened the nail is subjected to repeated minor traumata which may cause extension of the involved area and is accompanied by pain. The nail bed quickly becomes contaminated by bacteria or yeasts and there may be pus formation but often the infection is asymptomatic. Pseudomonas aeruginosa is a common contaminant and this will produce a characteristic coloration of the nail plate which may be green, blue or black (Plate **III** (*b*)) (Chernosky and Dukes, 1963).

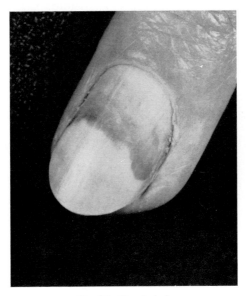

Fig. 85   Onycholysis

The condition is a very stubborn one and if not corrected the exposed nail bed becomes covered with keratin very similar to that of the finger tip and when this happens reattachment of the nail is very unlikely to occur.

The secondary infection is probably the main reason for the failure of the nail to reattach itself in the early stages. Ray (1963) recommends treatment of this by cutting away the loosened nail with sharp pointed nail clippers followed by the application of a 15% solution of sulphacetamide in 50% spirit to the nail bed. This is repeated daily whilst the nail has a chance to grow forward and reattach itself as it does so. Sulphacetamide 15% is bactericidal to all contaminants and also prevents the growth of fungi and yeasts. Wilson (1965) recommended 4% thymol in chloroform as a means of preventing infection and maceration of the nail bed. The author has found that some patients cannot tolerate 4% thymol and prefers 2% in chloroform. Both these methods are useful but neither is successful in every case. Sulphacetamide is applied with a brush but the thymol solution should be applied with cotton wool on an orange stick.

Dystrophia Mediana Canaliformis
(median nail dystrophy)

This is an uncommon condition of unknown aetiology first described by Heller (1928). It consists of a split or canal in the

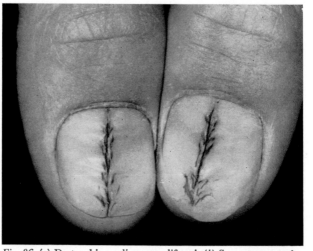

(a)

Fig. 86 (*a*) Dystrophia mediana canaliformis (*b*) Same, two months later (*c*) Same, another two months later showing spontaneous improvement

nail plate and is usually just off centre. Any finger nail may be involved but most often the thumb nails. The split starts at the cuticle and progresses to the free edge. There are usually a few feathery cracks extending laterally from the split towards, but not

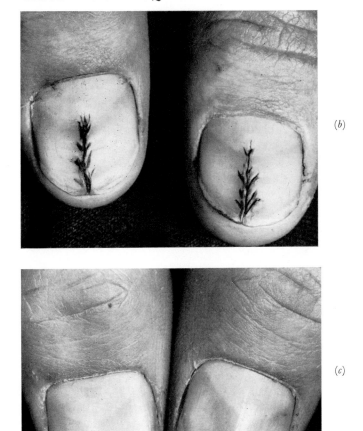

(b)

(c)

reaching, the edges of the nail. This has been likened to an inverted fir tree. After a period of months or years, the nail returns to normal in most cases but relapse may occur (Fig. 86). On healing, a ridge normally replaces the split. It is apparent that there is some temporary damage to the nail matrix and as most cases seem to have large half moons, so that a larger part of the

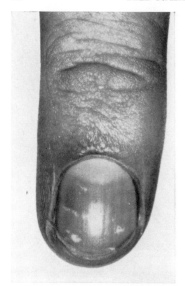

Fig. 87 Leukonychia punctata

Fig. 88 Leukony-
chia striata

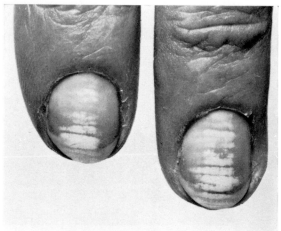

matrix is unprotected by the dorsal nail fold than usual, the damage may be of a traumatic nature. A few cases give a definite history of trauma. Familial cases have been recorded (Seller, 1974). Sutton (1965) described a case on a toe nail in which a flabby filament of fleshy tissue was present in the canal. He preferred the term 'solenonychia' for this deformity.

Treatment is usually unnecessary but protection from trauma is advised. The nail should be kept short to reduce the disability produced by a nail split into halves.

Diagnosis is generally obvious. A split as a result of definite trauma must be excluded as also must repeated trauma due to a habit tic and to splits as seen in the nail patella syndrome.

Leukonychia

This term is used to imply whitening of the nail plate itself. It may be congenital or acquired, partial or complete. The rare congenital leukonychia totalis is described on p. 174. Partial leukonychia is very common and may be punctate (Fig. 87) or striate (Fig. 88). It may occasionally be the result of illness, e.g. Mees' stripes in chronic arsenical poisoning, and has been described in association with many other diseases (Albright and

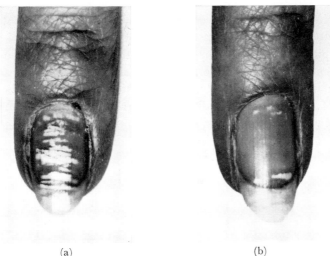

(a)   (b)

Fig. 89   (*a*) Traumatic leukonychia striata   (*b*) same nail 3 months later

Wheeler, 1964). In the great majority of punctate cases, however, which are extremely common, no cause can be found. Mitchell (1953) made an interesting study of his own nails over a period of one year and showed that some white spots appeared near the cuticle but others on other parts of the nail. Some disappeared before they reached the free edge and some increased in size after they had been formed.

In striate leukonychia a traumatic element is present in some cases and in particular overactive pushing back the cuticle in manicure. The condition will resolve if less active manicure is used (Fig. 89). There is no very satisfactory explanation for the whiteness but it may be due to incomplete keratinization so that nuclei or nuclear debris are retained in the nail plate.

Leukonychia must be distinguished from whitening due to other causes, e.g. fungal infection of the nail plate and whiteness of the nail bed in hypoalbuminaemia.

Leukonychia Striata Longitudinalis

Under this title, Higashi *et al.* (1971) described the occurrence in two patients of a white streak extending from cuticle to free margin and lasting for several years. In one case the white streak was attributed to the presence of abnormal cornified cells in the nail plate accompanied by parakeratotic hyperplasia of the nail bed epidermis and in the other to parakeratotic hyperplasia of the nail bed epidermis only. The condition was thought to be due to naevoid changes in the distal nail matrix below the white streak.

It would be difficult to differentiate this condition from white streaks in the nails in Darier's disease unless other evidence of that condition was present.

Parakeratosis Pustulosa

Under this heading Hjorth and Thomsen (1967) described a disorder confined to young children and especially girls. The lesions begin close to the free margin of the nail and in about 25% of cases a few isolated pustules or vesicles can be seen in the initial phase. These quickly clear and eczematoid changes cover the skin immediately adjacent to the free margin of the nail. The changes may extend to the dorsal nail fold or to the sides of finger or toe. The most striking and characteristic changes result

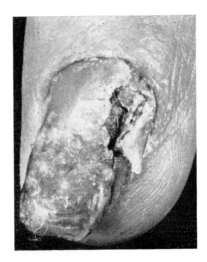

Fig. 90 Parakeratosis pustulosa

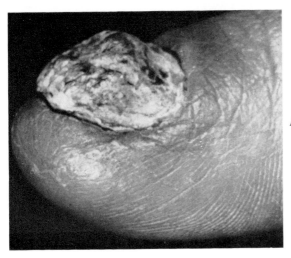

Fig. 91 Parakeratosis pustulosa

from hyperkeratosis under the free margin of the nail which rarely extends more than 1–2 mm into the nail bed. The nail itself is lifted and deformed and sometimes thickened. There may be pitting and rarely cross-ridging. The condition is more common on the hands and is usually limited to one digit, occasionally two, rarely more. On the hands the thumb and index finger are most often affected and on the feet, the great toes. The condition lasts a long time—often for a number of years—and may recur after apparent cure and may then affect a different digit. It does not, however, extend into adult life.

The author has seen a number of cases which would conform to this description (Figs. 90 and 91). The changes are at times very like psoriasis but Hjorth and Thomsen consider the condition to be an independent eczematoid eruption. Dulanto *et al.* (1974) and Botel *et al.* (1973) do not agree with this and suggest that it may be due to psoriasis, pustular psoriasis or eczema. Dulanto *et al.* give the histological findings in one case and they are indefinite.

Idiopathic Atrophy of the Nails

This is an uncommon condition. The nails are normal at birth but after a few years one or more nails become deformed.

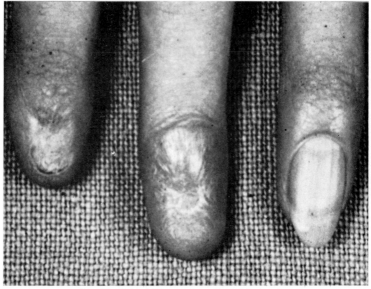

Fig. 92 Idiopathic atrophy—loss with scarring

The condition is progressive for a time but then becomes stationary but any damage is permanent. The changes vary from excessive ridging and opacity to pterygium formation and on some digits to total loss of the nail with scarring (Fig. 92). Finger nails are more often affected than toe nails. Although some patients appear to have poor peripheral circulation, this does not seem to be an important feature and the complete absence of pain or discomfort rules out an inflammatory process such as lichen planus. There are no skin lesions elsewhere (Samman, 1969). In one Negro family two sisters showed lesions very similar to one another.

Pterygium Inversum Unguis

Under this heading Caputo and Prandi (1973) described a patient who had an acquired abnormality in which the distal part of the nail bed remained adherent to the ventral surface of the nail plate thus eliminating the distal groove. It involved several fingers and there was no alteration of the nail plate. There was pain and bleeding if she attempted to cut the nails.

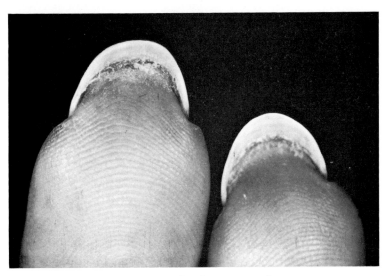

Fig. 93 Pterygium inversum unguis

A few similar reports have appeared subsequently. The author has seen a number of cases (Fig. 93) including one in whom two toes were affected.

Christophers (1975) describes under the heading *familial subungual pterygium* a mother and daughter who each had a condition of a similar nature which was also painful.

This type of change is not infrequently seen in patients with scleroderma of the progressive type, the result of local soft tissue atrophy.

Abnormalities of the Nails due to Drugs

The nails may be affected by drugs in various ways. Partial or total loss may result from a bullous eruption affecting the tips of

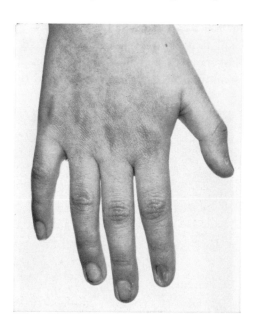

Fig. 94   Partial loss of nail following drug eruption

the digits. Any drugs which induce bullae, usually in the form of an erythema multiforme type of eruption, may be responsible. It is due to actual destruction of the nail matrix (Figs. 94 and 95).

Temporary loss has also been described as due to large doses of cloxacillin and cephaloridine (Eastwood *et al.*, 1969). Onycholysis due to the tetracyclines is described below.

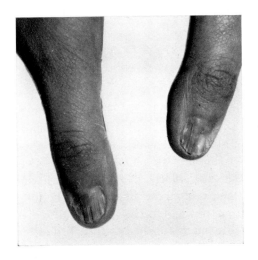

Fig. 95 Thumbs, same patient as in *Fig. 94*

There are a number of colours which are due to drugs. The nails may be stained a bluish colour with mepacrine and the nails will fluoresce yellow-green or white under Wood's light. Normal nails show a slight fluorescence of a violet-blue colour. Rarely prolonged tetracycline therapy will cause yellowing of the nails.

Chloroquine may produce a blue-black pigmentation of the nail beds (Tuffaneli *et al.*, 1963). Other antimalarials may produce bands of pigmentation longitudinal or vertical on the nail bed (Maguire, 1963; Colomb *et al.*, 1975). The fixed drug eruption of phenolphthalein if it occurs on the nail bed will produce a dark blue colour (Wise and Sulzberger, 1933). Argyria will discolour the nails a slate-blue. Inorganic arsenic can produce a longitudinal band of pigment or white stripes (Mees' stripes) across the nails (Mees, 1919).

Darkening of the nails has been noted by Pratt and Shanks (1974) following the administration of doxorubicin (Adriamycin) to white or coloured children for 6 weeks or longer. Pigmentation of skin and nails may be caused by hydroxyurea (Barety *et al.*, 1975).

Nail deformities and loss of hair are reported to be the cardinal signs of mercury poisoning from the use of hair bleaches. The bleach contained 5 to 6% of mercury and was marketed in Germany without statement of composition or warning of danger from its use (Wustner and Orfanos, 1975).

Photo-Onycholysis due to the Tetracyclines

Demethylchlortetracycline (Orentreich *et al.*, 1961) and much less often other tetracyclines (Frank *et al.*, 1971) induce a photosensitivity eruption which results in onycholysis of many digits. Strong sunlight is required to induce the change which is often accompanied by considerable discomfort. The author has seen one case in which the distal halves of all the affected nails became brown before separating from the nail beds. The condition is temporary so that the nails become reattached to their beds after a time.

Brittle Nails

As mentioned under symptomatology, brittle nails are very common and generally no cause can be found. The character of a nail varies considerably according to its water content. A normal nail contain about 18% water vapour. If this is greatly increased, e.g. after prolonged immersion in water, the nail becomes very soft. On the other hand, if it is considerably reduced the nail becomes brittle. This excess loss is liable to occur in a dry atmosphere and is equivalent to skin chapping. It is also liable to occur more rapidly if the nail is thin and if the nail is kept long so that there is more than the usual amount exposed to the atmosphere on upper and lower surfaces. It is not known how much of the moisture content of nail keratin is derived from the atmosphere and how much from the underlying soft tissues. Close attachment to the nail bed with the nails cut short to reduce the surface area exposed to the atmosphere will certainly restrict the amount of loss in a dry atmosphere. The brittleness is due to a lowered water content of the nail but the splitting which results from the brittleness is probably partly due to repeated increase and decrease of water content so that the nails change from soft to brittle frequently during the course of a day.

Treatment of brittle nails must be symptomatic. Avoidance of a very dry atmosphere and of frequent immersion of the hands in water is recommended. The nails should be kept trimmed as short as possible and the use of hand cream at night, especially one containing glycerin, may be helpful—e.g.

R. Salicylic acid ointment (2%)   } Equal parts
    Glycerin of starch

This should be applied regularly all over the finger tips. The use of nail varnish is not contraindicated.

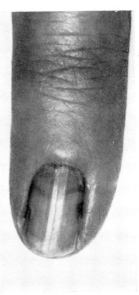

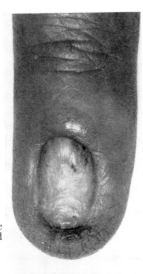

Fig. 96 Damage caused by weed killers

Fig. 97 Damage caused by weed killers

Damage Caused by Weed Killers

Samman and Johnston (1969) recorded cases of damage to finger nails resulting from contact with concentrated solution of paraquat and diquat. The material must have penetrated to the nail matrix and interfered with the growth of the nails. The changes ranged from white or brown bands across the base of the nails with softening of the nail plate to permanent loss of one nail (Figs. 96 and 97). Hearn and Keir (1971) have recorded similar damage following gross contamination with diluted solutions.

It seems probable that other chemicals which interfere with keratinization could produce a similar deformity if allowed to enter the posterior nail fold. The author has seen two patients who suffered severe damage from hydrofluoric acid. One patient had severe onycholysis (Plate III (d)) and the other partial destruction of thumb nails (Samman, 1977).

References

Albright, S D and Wheeler, C E (1964) Leukonychia. *Arch. Derm.* **90** 392

Baréty M, Audoly, P, Migozzi, B, Conil, J G and Dunjardin (1975) Pigmentation ungueale et cutanée au cours d'un traitment par hydroxy-urée *Bull. Soc. Fr. Derm. Syph.* **82** 208

Botela, R, Mascaro, J M, Martinez, C and Albero, F (1973) La parakeratosis pustulosa *Actas. Derm. Syph.* **64** 579

Caputo, R and Prandi, G (1973) Pterygium Inversum Unguis. *Arch. Derm.* **108** 817

Chernosky, M E and Dukes, C D (1963) Green nails. Importance of psuedomonas aeruginosa in onychia. *Arch. Derm.* **88** 548

Christophers, E (1975) Familial Subungual Pterygium *Der. Hautarzt* **26** 543

Colomb, D, Vittori, F, and Gho, A (1974) Pigmentation cutanéo-muqueuse et unguêale a la flavoquine. *Bull. Soc. Fr. Derm. Syph.* **82** 319

Dawber, R P R, Samman, P D and Bottoms, E (1971) Finger nail growth in idiopathic and psoriatic onycholysis. *Brit. J. Derm.* **85** 558

Dulanto, F de, Armigo-Moreno and Camacho-Martinez, F (1974) Parakeratosis Pustulose: Histological Findings, *Acta Dermatoven (Stock)* **54** 365.

Eastwood, J B, Curtis, J R, Smith, E K M and Wardener, H E de (1969) Shedding of nails apparently induced by the administration of large amount of cephaloridine and cloxacillin in two anephric patients. *Brit. J. Derm.* **81** 750

Frank, S B, Coher, H J and Minkin, W (1971) Photo-onycholysis due to tetracycline hydrochloride and doxycycline. *Arch. Derm.* **103** 520

Graciansky, P de and Boulle, S (1961) Association de koilonychie et de leuchonychie transmises en dominance. *Bull. Soc. Fr. Derm. Syph.* **68** 15

Heller, J (1928) Dystrophia unguium mediana canaliformis. *Dermat. Z.* **51** 416

Hearn, C E D and Keir, W (1971) Nail damage in spray operators exposed to Paraquat. *Brit. J. indust. Med.* **28** 399

Higashi, N, Sugai, T and Yamamoto T (1971) Leukonychia striata longitudi-nales. *Arch. Derm.* **104** 192

Hjorth, N and Thomsen, K (1967) Parakeratosis pustulosa. *Brit. J. Derm.* **79** 527

La Rossa, D and Hamilton, R (1971) Herpes simplex infections of the digits. *Arch. Surg.* **102** 600

Maguire, A (1962) Amodioquin hydrochloride; corneal deposits and pig-mented palate and nails after treatment of chronic discoid lupus erythema-tosus. *Lancet* **i** 667

Mees, R A (1919) Een Verschijnsel bij Polyneuritis Arsenicosa. *Nederl. T. Geneesh* **1** 391

Mitchell, J C (1953) A clinical study of leukonychia. *Brit. J. Derm.* **65** 121

Orentrich, N, Harber, L C and Tromovitch, T A (1961) Photosensitivity and photo-onycholysis due to demethylchlortetracycline. *Arch. Derm.* **83** 730

Pratt, C B and Shanks, E C (1974) Hyperpigmentation of the nail from doxo-rubicin (Adriamycin) *J. Amer. Med. Ass.* **228** 460

Ray, L (1963) Onycholysis. *Arch. Derm.* **88** 181

Samman, P D (1969) Idiopathic atrophy of the nails. *Brit. J. Derm.* **81** 746

Samman, P D (1977) Nail disorders caused by external influences. *J. Soc. Cosmet. Chem.* **28** 351

Samman, P D and Johnstone, E N M (1969) Nail damage associated with handling of paraquat and diquat. *Brit. med. J.* **1** 818

Seller, H (1974) Dystrophia Unguis Mediana canaliformis: familial occurrence *Hautarzt* **25** 456

Stern, H, Elek, S D, Millar, D N and Anderson, H F (1959) Herpetic whitlow. A form of cross-infection in hospitals. *Lancet* **ii** 871

Sutton, R L Jr. (1965) Solenonychia. *Sth. Med. J. Nashville* **58** 1143

Tuffanelli D, Abraham, R K and Dubois, E I (1963) Pigmentation from antimalarial therapy. *Arch. Derm.* **88** 419

Wilson, J W (1965) Paronychia and onycholysis. Etiology and therapy. *Arch. Derm.* **92** 726

Wise, F and Sulzberger, M B (1933) Drug eruptions: I Fixed phenolphthalein eruptions. *Arch. Derm.* **27** 549

Wustner, H and Orfanos, C E (1975) Nail changes and hair loss: cardinal signs of mercury poisoning from hair bleaches. *Dtsch. med. Wschr.* **100** 1694

Chapter 8

Nail Disorders Associated with Impaired Peripheral Circulation

The nail is easily damaged by reduction in its blood supply. It is in a vulnerable position, and cold by inducing vascular spasm may reduce the blood supply sufficiently to interfere with the formation of the nail plate. There are a number of ways in which the nail may react.

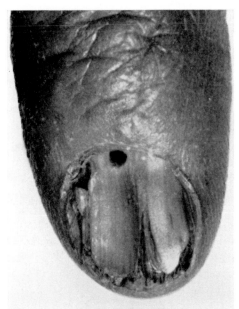

Fig. 98 Nail in patient with Raynaud's symptoms

Raynaud's symptoms of a number of years' duration will produce a rather characteristic deformity. The nail plate becomes thin and excessively ridged longitudinally (Fig. 98). Splits develop along the ridges and the thinning leads to brittleness of the nails and in some cases to flattening or koilonychia.

Partial onycholysis of one or more nails may occur. The thinning of the nail plate also allows the colour of the nail bed to show more clearly through the plate and makes the nail look redder than normal—this contrasts markedly with areas where onycholysis has occurred as these appear white (Plate IV (a) and (b)) or become dark through accumulation of dirt or due to secondary infection. The nails are usually kept short by the patient on account of their brittleness. Although the nails are of poor

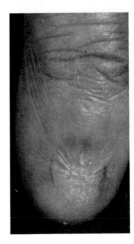

Fig. 99 Permanent loss of nail due to digital artery occlusion

quality the rate of growth is within normal limits but nearer the lower level of normal. Much less often, instead of becoming thinner the nails become thicker than normal. This change is often accompanied by onycholysis and the nail bed may become thick and rough. Secondary contamination by bacteria or candida may lead to darkening of the nail plate. This change is seen especially in old age and in diabetes.

Arteriograms on a number of patients have shown that spasm alone is sufficient to cause damage, although the same changes may occur in the presence of digital artery occlusion (Samman and Strickland, 1962; Strickland and Urquhart, 1963).

Permanent shedding of the nail with scarring is seen occasionally. This may be the result of digital artery occlusion when only

one (Fig. 99) or a few fingers are involved, but when many digits
are affected it may be the result of severe spasm without organic
damage to the vessels (Fig. 100).

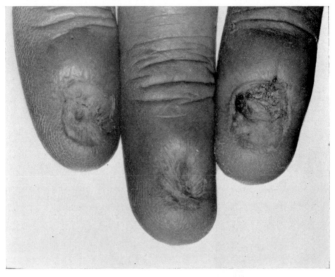

Fig. 100   Permanent loss of several nails associated with severe Raynaud's
symptoms but no arterial occlusion

Total or partial loss of one or more nails is not uncommon in
association with diabetes mellitus and arterial damage from
other causes including scleroderma (Fig. 101). Partial loss may
represent reduction in width or thickness of the nail.

Pterygium formation, the apparent overgrowth of the cuticle
and its fixation to the nail plate leading to closure of the nail
groove by fusion of the dorsal nail fold to the nail bed is described
by Edwards (1948) as characteristic of vasospasm and may
occasionally accompany the other changes described above
especially partial loss of the nails (Figs. 102 and 103). It is
doubtful however whether it is always due to arterial spasm, as it
may almost certainly accompany more permanent arterial
damage and is also seen at times in lichen planus and at other
times for no apparent cause.

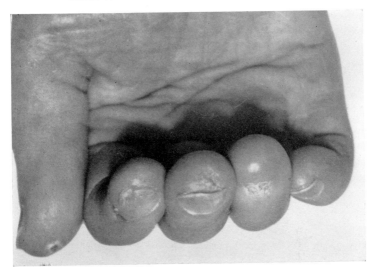

Fig. 101 Scleroderma—nail and soft tissue damage

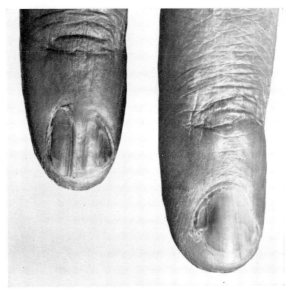

Fig. 102 Raynaud's symptoms—early pterygium formation

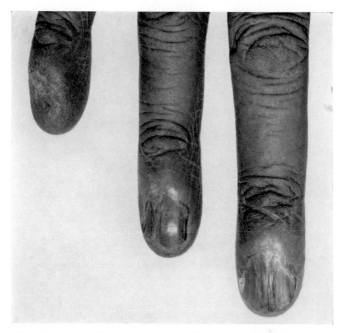

Fig. 103 Raynaud's symptoms—pterygium formation on two nails and
permanent loss of one nail with scarring

Onycholysis can occur as the only nail symptom of impaired circulation but more often is part of a symptom complex (Fig. 104).

Beau's lines may be seen as a result of excessive exposure to cold in persons who suffer from Raynaud's symptoms. Beau's lines consist of depressions on the nail surface and represent a temporary cessation of growth of the nails. They are encountered in a number of general medical disorders (see p. 112) when they affect all nails. Some nails are however likely to be spared when Beau's lines are induced by cold.

Chronic paronychia is very common in patients with cold hands and may complicate the pictures described above. Occasionally Candida albicans invades many nail plates and produces discoloration of the nails and, if onycholysis is present, it will produce thickening and irregularity of the nail beds. To the patient this is perhaps the most distressing effect of impaired circulation in the fingers.

The *treatment* of these disorders is the treatment of the underlying condition. The author has found inositol nicotinate 250 mg three or four times daily of considerable value in some cases. Unfortunately improvement is often only slight and other vasodilators may be preferred. Holti and Ingram (1963) described the treatment of chilblains with ultraviolet light and Holti in a personal communication has told me that he has had success in treating patients with nail dystrophies by this method. Patients

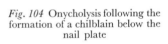

Fig. 104 Onycholysis following the formation of a chilblain below the nail plate

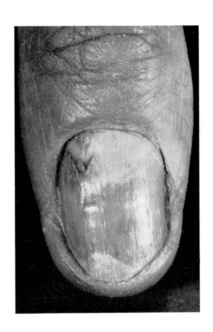

with impaired peripheral circulation and paronychia have been successfully treated and he has had some success in treating patients with psoriasis of the nails. The area treated is limited to the backs of the distal phalanges only. This part of the hand is very resistant to this form of irradiation so that a long exposure is required. Holti suggests 15 to 30 minutes at a distance of 25 to

30 cm from a powerful ultraviolet lamp. Three exposures are given one week apart and the dose should be increased by about 30% at second and third visits. The object is to produce a brisk erythema in 8 to 24 hours on each occasion. It is obviously wise to treat two fingers with lower dosage as a trial before exposing the others. The treatment should be given each year at the onset of cold weather for impaired circulation and whenever required for psoriasis. This treatment should be successful if spasm alone is responsible for the impaired circulation but if organic arterial blockage is present infusions of low molecular weight dextran (Rheomacrodex; Pharmacia) given two or three times a year or more often may be more useful (see Holti, 1965).

References

Edwards, E A (1948) Nail changes in functional and organic arterial disease. *New. Eng. J. Med.* **239** 362

Holti, G (1965) The effect of Intermittent Low Molecular Dextran upon the Digital Circulation in Systemic Sclerosis. *Brit. J. Derm.* **77** 560

Holti, G and Ingram, J T (1963) Physiotherapy in Dermatology. *Lancet* **i** 141

Samman, P D and Strickland, B (1962). Abnormalities of the finger nails associated with impaired peripheral blood supply. *Brit. J. Derm.* **74** 163

Strickland, B and Urquhart, W (1963) Digital arteriography, with reference to nail dystrophy. *Brit. J. Radiol.* **36** 465

Chapter 9

Nail Disorders attributed to or associated with other General Medical Conditions

Koilonychia

In this condition the nail loses its normal contour so that it becomes flat or truly concave (spoon-shaped) (Fig. 105).

It is the classical nail disorder of hypochromic (iron deficiency) anaemia. It is due to thinning and softening of the nail plates. Although usually confined to the fingers in anaemia, it may occur

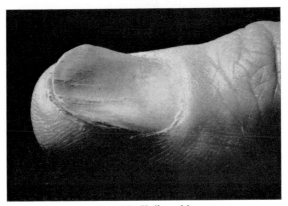

Fig. 105 Koilonychia

on the toes (Chatterjea, 1964). Jalili and Al-Kassab (1959) have shown that the sulphur-containing aminoacid cystime content of spoon-shaped nails is lower than normal so that iron deficiency *per se* is not the cause of the deformity. Nevertheless koilonychia can occur at times in the presence of low iron stores without actual anaemia (Beutler, 1964; Comaish, 1965).

Koilonychia is common in infants on finger and toe nails but is usually soon corrected. It occasionally persists into adult life and then represents a developmental anomaly (Hellier, 1950).

In a large Japanese family this was shown to be due to a single autosomal dominant gene (Handa *et al.*, 1960).

It is also seen on one or more fingers in association with the other changes described on p. 104 as occurring with Raynaud's symptoms. The separated halves of nails affected by pterygium formation may be spoon-shaped, as also may the two halves of split nails in the nail patella syndrome (p. 167).

Occasionally it occurs as an occupational disorder probably as the result of softening with oils or soaps, it is not uncommon in motor mechanics (Dawber, 1974). It has been recorded on the toes of ricksha boys in South Africa as a result of trauma (Bentley-Phillips and Bayles, 1971).

In iron deficiency with or without anaemia the administration of iron will soon correct the deformity. An explanation for the shaping of spoon nails is given on p. 116.

Beau's Lines

These are associated with any severe disability which temporarily interferes with the rate of growth of the nail, including

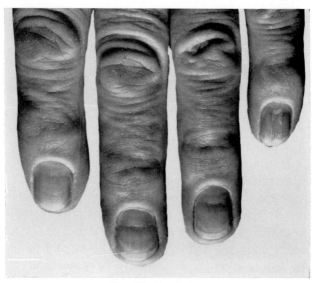

Fig. 106   Beau's lines

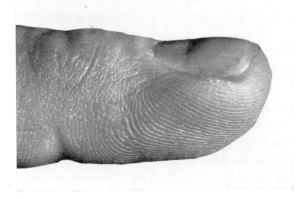

Fig. 107 Beau's lines—side view

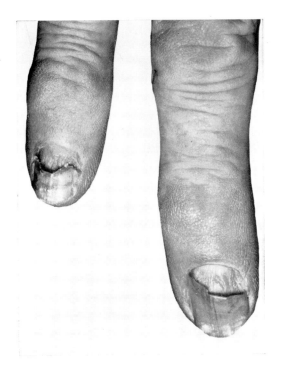

Fig. 108 Beau's lines—severe and leading to temporary loss of the nail

measles, mumps, pneumonia and coronary thrombosis. Beau's report dates back to 1846. The condition is represented by a depression on the surface of all nails, (Figs. 106 and 107). It does not show up for some weeks after the damage has been inflicted and then moves forward with the growth of the nail. By this time the rate of the nail growth has returned to normal.

If the interference with the nutrition of the nail is severe the depression may extend right through the nail plate and lead to temporary shedding of the nail (Fig. 108). Probably the only condition which interferes with the rate of growth of the nail in young persons with any regularity is measles (Sibinga, 1959). When lines appear on isolated nails the aetiology is unlikely to be due to any general disturbance but to local causes. They are seen occasionally after exposure to extreme cold in patients with Raynaud's symptoms. They are also found at times after local injury or in association with the carpal tunnel syndrome. Similar lines are seen with dermatitis but here they are more irregular and may be repeated on the affected nails.

Onycholysis

This has come to be associated with thyroid disorders, both hypo-(Fox, 1940) and hyper-thyroidism (Luria and Asper, 1958). It is, however, found in many other conditions and is one of the commonest nail symptoms. Other causes are listed on p. 20.

Finger Clubbing
(hippocratic nails)

Simple clubbing is classically associated with lung disease or heart disease with cyanosis. At an early stage of development the slight change at the finger ends may be hard to recognise as it consists only of loss of the normal angle between the nail and the posterior nailfold. Later the distal phalanx becomes enlarged and there may be an increase in the size of the nail (Fig. 109). A more severe form known as hypertrophic pulmonary osteoarthropathy is characterised by periostitis affecting the metacarpals, the two proximal rows of phalanges and the terminal few inches of ulna and radius in the hands and arms and corresponding bones in the feet and legs. The great majority of these cases are due to bronchogenic carcinoma.

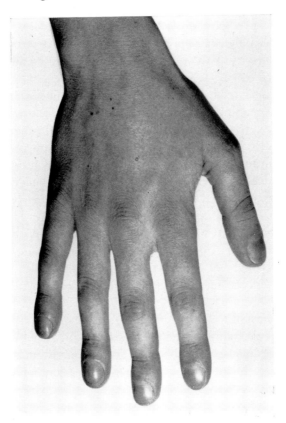

Fig. 109   Finger clubbing

A third form (Stone 1975) is known as pachydermo-periostosis. It is rare and generally considered idiopathic. In addition to clubbing there is a spade like enlargement of the hands. Thickening of legs and forearms involving bone and soft tissue and thickening of facial tissues. It affects especially adolescent males and is self limiting.

Clubbing also occurs in some cases of thyroid disease and in a number of abdominal conditions including biliary cirrhosis, sprue and ulcerative colitis. It has been suggested that it occurs only in disease of the organs supplied by the vagus nerve (Young, 1966); thus in ulcerative colitis clubbing occurs only if the disease affects that part of the colon which is supplied by the vagus. Although usually an important physical sign it is occasionally present from birth without any underlying disease and it may be familial.

The factors involved in the development of finger clubbing are obscure and no single cause will explain every case. Arteriograms show that there is abundant blood flow through the digits and this may be the result of opening up of arteriovenous anastomoses. The fault in many cases may lie in the lungs which normally act as a detoxicating agent for venous blood. When clubbing is present mixed arterial and venous blood is shunted past normal lung tissue and escapes its detoxicating action. Hall (1959) suggests that the substance present in venous blood which is responsible for the opening up of arteriovenous anastomoses is reduced ferritin. On oxidation by passing through normal lung tissue it becomes inert. Finger clubbing has been discussed in leading articles in the 'Lancet' (1959 and 1975) and the 'British Medical Journal' (1977).

Stone and Maberry (1965) and Stone (1975) put forward an hypothesis to explain the abnormal shape of nails in clubbing and koilonychia. They suggest that nail formation follows simple structural rules. Nail is much like a sheet of plastic being extruded from a press. It is shaped by the soft tissue that surrounds it during the period of keratinisation. They consider that there must be some common mechanism for the formation of clubbed and spoonshaped nails. The diverse disorders which will produce these changes are more likely to have an effect on connective tissue than on hard keratin.

Nail changes in spooning and clubbing are the result of an angulation of the (principal) matrix secondary to connective tissue changes. Spooning occurs if the distal end of the matrix is relatively low compared with proximal end and clubbing if the distal end is relatively high compared with the proximal end. In severe anaemia the distal end may be depressed below its normal level due to anoxia and atrophy of the distal connective tissue. In clubbing there is an increase in volume of the distal phalanx due to connective tissue proliferation and at times due to increased vascular flow. This will result in the distal end of the matrix being elevated.

Colour Changes

White nails have been described by Terry (1954A) in association with hepatic cirrhosis. The colour change is not in the nail itself but is apparently the result of changes in the nail bed. It is therefore quite different from leukonychia. In severe cases all finger nails are affected and the nails exhibit a ground-glass-like opacity of almost the entire nail bed. There may be a zone of normal pink near the distal edge of the nail. The reason for the pallor is so far unexplained. In some cases the white area may be peaked distally (Morey and Burke, 1955).

Paired narrow white bands have been described by Muehrcke (1956) in patients with chronic hypoalbuminaemia (Fig. 110). These bands run parallel with the lunula and are separated from one another and from the lunula by areas of normal pink nail. They apparently do not move forward with the nail and therefore cannot be in the nail plate. They disappear if the serum albumin level is restored to normal but recur on relapse. The reason for their formation is unexplained and they are by no means always present in hypoalbuminaemia.

Red half-moons were described by Terry (1954B) in association with congestive heart failure.

Azure half-moons were noted by Bearn and McKusick (1958) in two patients with hepato-lenticular degeneration (Wilson's disease). The colour change was restricted to the lunulae and is beautifully illustrated in two colour photographs.

The half-and-half nail was described by Lindsay (1967) in renal disease and azotaemia. In this condition the proximal nail bed is white and the distal half red, pink or brown. Leyded and Wood (1972) showed that the pigment is melanin and suggest that the

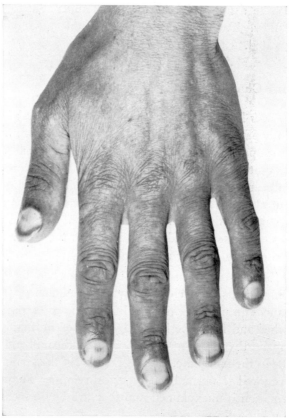

Fig. 110 White nails in patient convalescent from chronic hypoalbuminaemia (polycystic kidneys)

cause is due to the stimulation of the melanocytes in the nail matrix by sudden renal decompensation. Brown nail-bed arcs and chronic renal disease are described by Stewart and Raffle (1972).

Expedition nails. Juel-Jensen (1975) points out that persons suffering semi-starvation whilst on expedition develop white bands on their nails corresponding in width to the period of deprivation. The condition is probably due to protein deficiency.

In addition to these rather specific changes, it should be remembered that the nails look pale in any severe anaemia. Colour changes due to drugs are described on p. 99.

Pigmented bands on nails: Dark brown or black pigmented bands running in the long axis of the nail have been described as a sign of malnutrition in India by Bisht and Singh (1962). However, pigmented bands are very common in coloured persons as a result of trauma so that their importance as a sign of malnutrition is probably small (see p. 128).

The Yellow Nail Syndrome

This is the name given by Samman and White (1964) to a rather characteristic condition. The patients notice that their nails cease, or almost cease, to grow and some months later take on a yellow or greenish colour (Plate IV (*a*)). The nails normally remain smooth and may be somewhat thickened. They may be excessively curved from side to side, the lateral margins are less covered by soft tissue than in normal nails, and the cuticle is usually deficient (Fig. 111). One or more nails may show a distinct hump (Plate IV (*d*)). In a few cases there are ridges across the nails indicating variations in their rate of growth but overall the rate of growth is very slow, being reduced to 0.25 mm per week or less compared with 0.5 mm, the lower limit of normal. In some months there may be no measurable growth at all. Onycholysis often affects one or more nails and may extend so far towards the matrix that the nail plate is shed. It is very slowly replaced.

In addition to the changes in the nails themselves, there is usually some oedema. This may be confined to the finger tips but is often more widespread. The ankles are often swollen and there may be oedema of the face. Very severe oedema is seen

occasionally. Lymphangiograms may show changes in the lymphatic vessels as seen in primary lymphoedema, namely atresia, or
a single varicose lymphatic may replace the normal sized vessels.
However, in some patients even with severe oedema clinically, the
vessels appear normal on lymphangiography. This suggests that
there may be a fuctional as well as an anatomical abnormality.

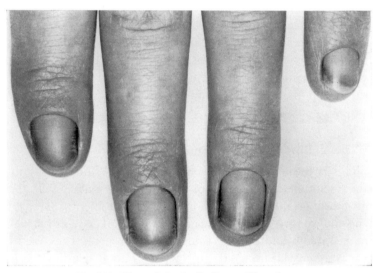

Fig. 111   The nails in the "yellow nail" syndrome

Many patients also have some chest symptoms. Chronic
bronchitis is most common but bronchiectasis (Dilley *et al.*, 1968)
is not infrequent and pleural effusions are found occasionally
(Emerson, 1966). Hiller *et al.* (1972) describe pulmonary com-
plications in 12 patients. Eight had recurrent pleural effusion,
5 had bronchiectasis and pleural effusion. Three of these 5 also
had sinusitis. They also noted that patients with the yellow nail
syndrome were liable to develop malignant neoplasms. It seems
probable that the lymphatic abnormality plays some part in the
production of these changes. Abnormalities of lymphatics in
other viscera, e.g. the gastrointestinal tract, are encountered
much less often.

Treatment of this disorder is unrewarding. Quite often with supportive treatment the nails improve in appearance for $\frac{1}{3}$ to $\frac{1}{2}$ of the distance from cuticle to free edge, whilst the distal portion remains discoloured. Complete spontaneous recovery in the appearance of the nails has been seen occasionally. Partial or complete recovery occurs in about 30% of patients but there may be a relapse. The improvement in the appearance of the nails is accompanied by a return to normal rate of growth of the nails.

Shell Nail Syndrome Associated with Bronchiectasis

Cornelius and Shelley (1967) describe under this heading the case of a patient who, following whooping cough at the age of four years, developed bronchiectasis and at the age of five changes in the finger nails were noted. All showed longitudinal curvature and there was dystrophy of the finger tip resulting from atrophy of the distal nail bed. X-ray of one finger showed thinning of the distal phalanx and complete loss of tufting. The nail plate could be seen to be separated from the nail bed. There seems to be little difference between this condition and some cases of the yellow nail syndrome.

Splinter Haemorrhages

Since the early report by Horder (1920), splinter haemor- rhages below the nails have come to be associated with subacute bacterial endocarditis. They occur, however, in many other medical conditions including trichinosis (when they are said to be transverse instead of in the long axis of the nail), severe rheuma- toid arthritis, uninfected mitral stenosis, peptic ulceration, hypertension and malignant neoplasms (Kuske, 1961). They are also commonly seen in psoriasis, dermatitis and fungal infec- tion of the nails. Splinter haemorrhages may also be the result of minor trauma as shown by the fact that patients recently admitted to hospital more often show splinter haemorrhages than patients who have been in hospital for some weeks (Gross and Tall, 1963).

The symptom is thus so common that its importance as a sign of disease is not great.

Ridging and Beading

These have been shown by Hamilton (1960) to occur more often in patients with rheumatoid arthritis than in normal subjects. Regular longitudinal ridging sometimes with a beaded appearance is much commoner in old age than in youth, but Hamilton claims that in all ages above 30 it is commoner in patients with rheumatoid arthritis than in normal controls. The fact that it occurs in quite a high proportion of normal people (Fig. 112) makes it doubtful if its occurrence in rheumatoid arthritis is of any great significance.

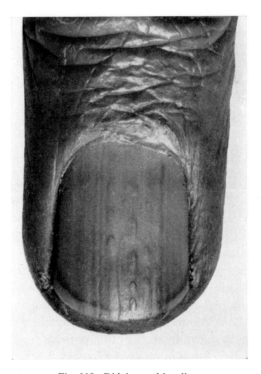

Fig. 112   Ridging and beading

The Senile Nail

Under this heading, Lewis and Montgomery (1955) describe the changes seen in many but by no means all elderly persons. The condition affects both fingers and toes. The nails appear dull and opaque and present longitudinal ridging. The colour varies from shades of yellow or green to grey. The thickness of the nail may be normal or it may be increased or decreased. There is an increased tendency to split into layers and growth of the nail is slow.

Histologically, changes in the nail bed consist of thickening of the walls of the blood vessels and merging of elastic and connective tissues in the cutis. These changes may be due in part to solar damage, the nail plate tending to amplify the effect of sunlight on the tissues immediately below it.

Paraneoplastic Acrokeratosis of Bazex

Baran (1977) in a letter to the Archives of Dermatology draws attention to this condition which is due to a carcinoma of the upper respiratory or digestive tract.

This condition begins suddenly and affects the nails first. The nails are deformed by subungual hyperkeratosis which pushes up the free edge. The surface is irregular and flaky and the nails may actually be destroyed. The condition resembles severe psoriatic deformity. The digits are covered with rough, fissured and keratotic patches. There may be paronychia. The condition may clear if the carcinoma is removed.

References

Baran, R (1977) Paraneoplastic Acrokeratosis of Bazex *Arch. Derm.* **113** 1613

Bearn, A G and McKuisck, V A (1958) Azure lunulae. *J. Amer. med. Ass.* **166** 904

Beau, J H S (1846) Certain caractères de semeliologie retrospective, présentes par les ongles. *Arch. Gen. med.* **9** 447

Bentley-Phillips, B and Bayles, M A H (1971) Occupational Koilonychia of the toe nails. *Brit. J. Derm.* **85** 140

Beutler, E (1964) Tissue effects of iron deficiency. In Gross, F (Ed.) Iron Metabolism. Springer-Verlag. Berlin. Gottingen. Heidelberg

Bischt, D B and Singh, S S (1962) Pigmented bands on nails. A new sign of malnutrition. *Lancet* **i** 507

British Medical Journal, Leading article (1977) Finger clubbing and hypertrophic pulmonary osteoarthropathy. *Brit. Med. J.* **3** 785

Chatterjea, J B (1964) Some aspects of iron-deficiency anaemia in India. In Gross, F (Ed.) Iron Metabolism. Springer-Verlag. Berlin. Gottingen, Heidelberg

Comaish, J S (1965) Diseases of Nails. *Newcastle med. J.* **28** 253

Cornelius, C E III and Shelley, W B (1967) Shell nail syndrome associated with bronchiectasis. *Arch. Derm.* **96** 694

Dawber, R (1974) Occupational Koilonychia. *Brit. J. Derm* **91** Supplement 10 11

Dilley, J J, Kierland, R R, Randall, R V and Shick, A M (1968) Primary lymphedema associated with yellow nails and pleural effusions. *J. Amer. med. Ass.* **204** 122

Emerson, P A (1966) Yellow nails, lymphoedema and pleural effusions. *Thorax* **21** 247

Fox, E C (1940) Diseases of the nails. Report of cases of onycholysis. *Arch. derm.* **41** 98

Gross, N J and Tall, R (1963) Clinical significance of splinter haemorrhages. *Brit. med. J.* **2** 1496

Hall, G H (1959) The cause of digital clubbing. Testing a new hypothesis. *Lancet* **i** 750

Hamilton, E D B (1960) Nail studies in rheumatoid arthritis. *Ann. rheum. Dis.* **19** 167

Handa, Y, Handa, K, Koaka, S and Mitani, S (1960) A note in the genetics of koilonychia. *Acta. Genet. med. Gemell* **9** 309

Hellier F F (1960) Hereditary koilonychia. *Brit. J. Derm.* **62** 213

Hiller E, Rosenow, E C and Olsen, A M (1972) Pulmonary manifestations of the yellow nail syndrome. *Chest* **61** 452

Horder, T (1920) Discussion on clinical significance and course of subacute bacterial endocarditis. *Brit. med. J.* **2** 301

Jalili, M A and Al-Kassab, S (1959) Koilonychia and cystine content of nails. *Lancet* **ii** 108

Juel-Jensen B E (1975) Expedition nails. *Brit. med. J.* **2** 140

Kuske H von (1961) Splitterblutungen des Nagelplatte. *Dermatologica* **123** 219

Lancet Leading article (1959) Clubbing of the fingers and Osteoarthropathy *Lancet* **ii** 390

Lancet. Leading article (1975) Finger clubbing. *Lancet* **i** 1285

Leyded, J J & Wood, M G (1972) The half and half nail of uremic onychodystrophy. *Arch. Derm.* **105** 591

Lindsay, P G (1967) The half-and-half nail. *Arch. Intern. Med.* **119** 583

Luria, M N and Asper, S P Jr. (1958) Onycholysis in hyperthyroidism. *Ann. intern. Med.* **49** 102

Morey, D A J and Burke J O (1955) Distinctive nail changes in advanced hepatic cirrhosis. *Gastroenterology* **29** 258

Muehrcke, R C (1956) The finger nails in chronic hypoalbuminaemia. *Brit. med. J.* **1** 1327

Samman, P D and White, W F (1964) The yellow nail syndrome. *Brit. J. Derm.* **76** 53

Sibinga, M S (1959) Observations on growth of finger nails in health and disease. *Pediatrics* **24** 225

Stewart, W K and Raffle, E J (1972) Brown nail-bed arcs and chronic renal disease. *Brit. med. J.* **1** 784

Stone, O J (1975) Spoon nails and clubbing. Significance and mechanisms. *Cutis.* **16** 235

Stone, O J and Maberry, J D (1965) Spoon nails and clubbing. Review and possible mechanisms. *Tex. St. J. Med.* **61** 620

Terry, R (1954A) White nails in hepatic cirrhosis. *Lancet* **i** 757

Terry, R (1954B) Red half-moons in cardiac failure. *Lancet* **ii** 842

Young, J R (1966) Ulcerative colitis and finger-clubbing. *Brit. med. J.* **1** 278

Chapter 10

Nail Deformities Due to Trauma

A great many nail deformities are the result of trauma and trauma may affect the nails in many ways. In this chapter, therefore, a number of otherwise unrelated conditions are discussed.

The damage inflicted on the nail may be the result of a single or occasional injury, or it may be the result of constantly repeated minor injuries. The first type will be described as acute trauma and will produce permanent damage to the nail if the matrix area is injured. Repeated minor injuries will be described as chronic trauma.

ACUTE TRAUMA

Haematomata

These are probably the commonest occasional injuries inflicted on the nail (Fig. 113). The amount of damage varies greatly and in severe cases is accompanied by much pain. Whether or not the haemorrhage is immediately apparent depends on the location of the injury. If it is under the exposed nail the bleeding will be immediately apparent but if the injury is below the dorsal nail fold the haemorrhage may not be visible for 2 or 3 days and will then move forward with the growth of the nail. Stone and Mullins (1963) have shown that a haemorrhage in the matrix area is incorporated into the nail plate, whilst one distal to the lunula remains subcuticular unless removed. In the majority of cases of severe damage, partial or total temporary shedding of the nail occurs if the blood is not released very quickly. Most patients request treatment for the relief of pain. The pain is produced by the increasing pressure below the nail. Reduction of pressure is best carried out by making a small puncture hole through the nail plate with a hot cautery point or other suitable instrument

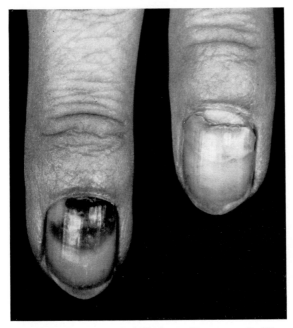

Fig. 113 Haematoma of middle finger. Temporary shedding of index finger nail following trauma but without haematoma formation

without local anaesthesia. This procedure not only relieves the pain but may save the nail. The possibility of an underlying fracture must be considered. In a series described by Farrington (1964) this was present in 19%.

Splits and Ridges

Permanent splits will result from any acute trauma which severs the matrix area (Fig. 114). The associated injuries are usually more severe and the damage to the nail is not appreciated for some months. It is then observed that the nail is split throughout its length, into two or more portions. If the damage is reported soon after the injury it may be possible to repair it by removing the nail plate and putting in sutures to pull together the separated parts of the matrix. If successful, the split will be replaced by a ridge down the nail. Unfortunately, it is often not for some

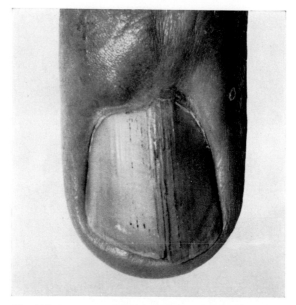

Fig. 114 Permanent ridging and splitting of nail following
trauma

months or years after the injury that the damage is reported. In
these cases plastic repair may be possible by removing permanently the smaller portion and recentering the remainder (see
Johnson, 1971). Sometimes the patient has difficulty in recalling
the accident which may have appeared quite minor at the time,
but proved sufficient to produce permanent damage to the matrix.

Permanent ridges on isolated nails are produced by similar
injuries to those producing splits, but of lesser degree.

Pigment Bands

Bands of pigmentation may often form in the nail plate after
minor injuries in patients with heavily pigmented skin. A sewing
machine needle run through the finger at the level of the nail
matrix is readily recalled by the patient (Fig. 115), but much less
damage may produce the same effect. The resulting pigment
bands may be temporary or permanent. In the white races,

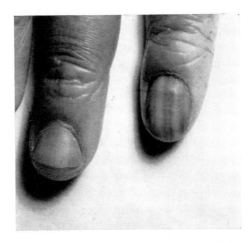

Fig. 115 Pigmented bands on nail plate following injury with sewing machine needle

bands of pigment appear on the nail plate much less often and in these people may be the result of an active junctional naevus in the matrix area (p. 156).

Other Deformities

It is not uncommon to see a patient with a partially amputated finger tip with a severely distorted nail often short and thick, the end result of an injury to the finger. Great hypertrophy of the nail is occasionally the result of a single injury but more often is the result of repeated trauma (p. 145).

CHRONIC TRAUMA

It will be seen that there are several ways in which repeated trauma may be inflicted. Nail biting, cuticle biting, and playing with the nails or cuticles are all common habits which may produce considerable damage to the nails. Ill-fitting footwear, especially in children, will lead to many nail deformities of the toes. Injuries from chemicals or friction at work or in the home may result in damage in various ways, whilst the use of nail varnish may occasionally produce staining of the nails which cannot easily be removed. Frequent immersion of the hands in water is a more subtle form of injury but is probably the most important factor in the splitting of the nail into layers.

Nail Biting and Cuticle Biting

These very common habits may produce great distortion of the nail. The patients will usually freely admit to the habit but occasionally the patient will claim that his deformity is due to lack of growth of the nail. This can easily be disproved by putting a fixed dressing on one finger for a few weeks or by making a small mark on one nail near the half-moon and watching it move to the tip a few weeks later. Bitten nails in fact are said to grow rather faster than normal. Bitten nails are usually very short and irregular (Figs. 116 and 117). The patient spends much time biting off spicules formed at an earlier session of biting. Cuticle biting is similar and may result in recurrent attacks of paronychia usually of a minor nature. Some people may bite only one nail and then only in times of stress such as watching an exciting television

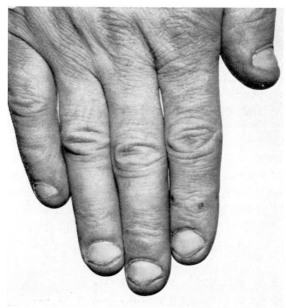

Fig. 116 Bitten nails

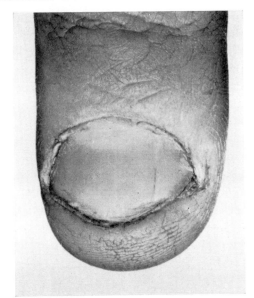

Fig. 117 Close-up of one finger
shown in *Fig. 116*

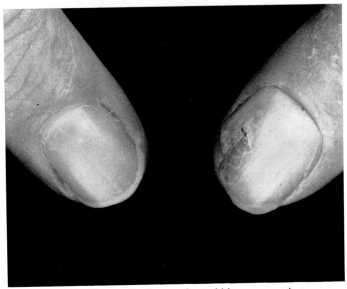

Fig. 118   Bitten nail—damage due to biting over matrix area

programme. The biting in these cases may be away from the tip and may even encroach on the matrix area, when an entirely different deformity will be produced (Fig. 118). If the damage produced by biting is severe the patient may further aggravate the condition by picking off small pieces constantly so that there may be apparent total loss of the nail. An occlusive dressing applied to the finger tip will prevent further damage and permit regrowth of a normal nail (Samman, 1977). In any case of finger nail deformity otherwise unexplained, it is always worth enquiring about nail biting. Rarely, the reverse occurs and one nail is spared whilst the remainder are bitten (Fig. 119).

Deformities very similar to nail biting can be caused by picking at the nail or by very close trimming.

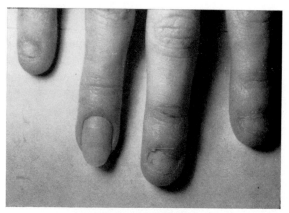

Fig. 119   Nail biting—one nail spared

Treatment of nail biting is very unsatisfactory. The answer is so obvious but the patient often cannot be persuaded to give up the habit. If one parent nail bites, the children are more likely to be nail biters than otherwise and it may prove more easy to reason with the parent than with the child. Periungual warts are an important complication of nail biting. The treatment of these is discussed on p. 151.

Hang Nails

Hang nails are very common in nail biters but may also result from many other forms of injury incurred in the home or at work. They consist of small portions of horny epidermis which have split away from the lateral nail fold. They may extend deep enough to expose the underlying cutis when they will be painful and may be the site of origin of bacterial infection. They are best treated by cutting away with very sharp pointed scissors. If infection is present, an antiseptic paint should be applied.

The Habit Tic of Playing with the Nails

This is another but less common habit (Samman, 1963) and often produces a rather characteristic deformity. The damage is usually inflicted on one or both thumb nails by one of the fingers

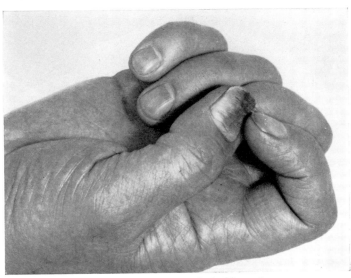

Fig. 120 Habit tic—method of formation

of the same hand. The finger is placed on the dorsal nail fold and then drawn forward over the nail plate (Fig. 120) and the process is repeated frequently. The damage is caused partly by this and partly by picking at the cuticle. The cuticle will be seen to be pulled away from the nail (Macaulay, 1966).

Less often, a finger of the opposite hand is used to pick at the cuticle. The resulting damage usually takes the form of a depression about 2 mm wide down the centre of the nail from the cuticle to the tip and from it extend a number of cross ridges almost to the edges of the nail (Fig. 121). The depression is not always present and may be present on one thumb nail and absent from the other. When the depression is absent, the cross ridging is the

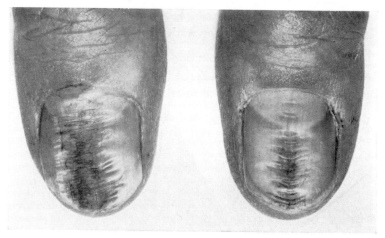

Fig. 121 Traumatic nail dystrophy due to a habit tic

only visible sign. The presence or absence of a depression probably depends on the force used by the finger which produces the damage. In a few cases a finger other than the thumb carries the deformity and in these cases it is the thumb which does the damage. The patient is usually well aware of his habit tic, but is surprised when the cause of his deformity is explained to him. Like nail biting, the habit is very difficult to break once established.

The only conditions likely to be mistaken for this deformity are the true median dystrophy (dystrophia mediana canaliformis of Heller) which is described on p. 90, dermatitis affecting the nail and trauma inflicted by other means. In dermatitis the cross ridges are less regular than in the habit tic and there is likely to be evidence of dermatitis on the finger or a recent history of dermatitis. In the median dystrophy there is a true split down the nail and the lateral projections are of a feathery appearance. Occasionally cross ridging is the result of overactive pushing back of the cuticle during manicuring (Fig. 122) or it may be the result of repeated intense pressure on the tip of the nail.

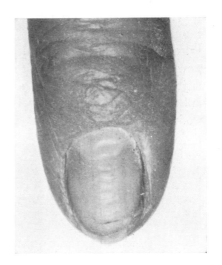

Fig. 122 Minor ridging due to pushing back of cuticles

The condition will right itself if the patient gives up the habit or if an occlusive dressing is applied over the affected finger for a sufficient time.

Nut-Cracker's Nails

This title was used to describe nail splitting and onycholysis in a patient who separated the two halves of cracked walnuts with his nails over a period of 10 years (Cohen *et al.*, 1975).

Onychotillomania

A few cases of this deformity have been seen by the author. It was described by Combes and Scott (1951). Essentially it is similar to the habit tic but aetiologically is closer to parasito-phobia. The patient picks off small pieces of nail and fragments of skin from the surrounding nail fold and may claim that they contain parasites. A rough and irregular nail and nail fold results. Many finger nails are involved.

Nail Artefacts

These fortunately are rare. They are produced by deliberate trauma and take various forms. Piercing the nail with a sharp instrument in the region of the half-moon interferes with nail growth locally and, as a result of sepsis, granulation tissue may project through the nail. In another form the patient inserts a nail file or other instrument under the cuticle and by so doing produces a chronic or acute paronychia (Fig. 123). Several

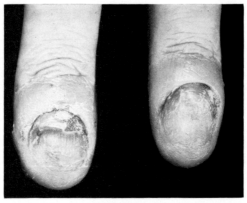

Fig. 123 Paronychia, deliberately produced

fingers or toes may be involved. The patient will gain some benefit from the injury.

Splitting into Layers
(lamellar dystrophy)

This is a very common complaint among women. The nails do not split along ridges longitudinally but horizontally through the thickness of the nail so that portions of the surface break off near the free margin (Fig. 124). Many forms of trauma probably contribute to the cause of this complaint, but the most important may be the repeated uptake and drying out of water.

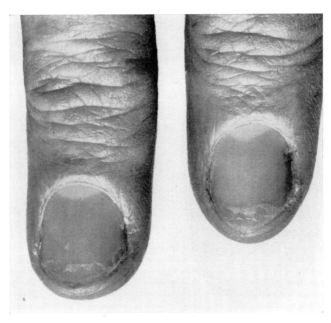

Fig. 124   Splitting of nails into layers

When immersed in water, especially if alkaline, the nail quickly becomes soft through the taking up of excess water, but this excess is quickly lost again on exposure to a dry atmosphere. This repeated wetting and drying leads to a lack of adhesion between the cells of the nail plate and splits develop. These splits can easily be shown to exist microscopically before the patient becomes aware of the damage they may cause. Although common in women, this condition is seldom seen in men. There are probably a number of reasons why this is so. Firstly, women like to keep their nails longer than men so that there is more free margin with both surfaces exposed to the atmosphere and therefore wetting and drying occur more rapidly. Secondly, women more often have their hands in water than men. Thirdly, nail varnish and varnish removers and excess manicuring may be of some importance aetiologically and, finally, women are more conscious of their nails than men and are therefore more likely to report the defect. The condition is more common in winter than in summer, probably because in winter the atmosphere is drier.

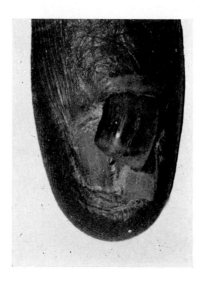

Fig. 125 Trauma has split the nail into two layers

Treatment is unfortunately unsatisfactory. The patient should be instructed to avoid excess wetting as far as possible and to keep her nails as short as she will tolerate. Nail varnish should not be forbidden because this at least covers the defect to some extent. Oily removers should however be recommended. The author has not found calcium or gelatin to be of any real value in treatment. A good nail hardener is needed but one which is free from irritants or sensitisers such as formaldehyde.

Very occasionally a single nail is encountered which is split into two layers throughout its length (Fig. 125). This is different from lamellar dystrophy and is the result of a single injury splitting the matrix. This is sometimes called *onychoschizia*.

Cutaneous Microwave Injury

Under this heading Brodkin and Bleiberg (1975) described nail deformities in two patients who were operating a microwave oven which was probably faulty. The damage consisted of deep cross ridges on the nails of the fingers which opened and closed the oven. The patients suffered no discomfort.

Damage caused by Nail Cosmetics

Although nail cosmetics are very well tolerated in most cases, they can cause damage or disfigurement in a number of ways.

Staining of the nails from nail varnish. Some pigments which are used as tints for nail varnish tend to leak out of the varnish and penetrate the nail. The colour of the pigment may be quite different from the finished product so that a red varnish may stain the nails yellow. This can be disconcerting to the patient and the pigment is too deep in the nail to be removed. It grows out with the nail and no active treatment is required. No permanent injury is caused. Cosmetic firms are aware of this danger but some popular tints are difficult to obtain without the use of one of the less reliable dyes (see Calnan, 1967). There are a number of different pigments which can cause this type of staining (Samman, 1977).

Stick-on nail dressings. Although dermatitis of the eyelids and sides of the neck is not infrequently caused by nail varnish, it is very uncommon to see dermatitis near the nails from this cause. The average nail varnish is well tolerated and appears to cause little damage to the nails.

For a short time, however, there were marketed in this country and in the United States synthetic stick-on nail dressings which had a number of advantages over varnish such as ease and speed of application. Unfortunately, it soon became apparent that they were causing much damage to the nails and had to be withdrawn from public use. It seems most likely that the reason for the damage was that the material was imporous and interfered with the free exchange of moisture between the nail plate and the atmosphere (Samman, 1961). On removal, fine portions of nail remained attached to the adhesive of the nail dressing and the nail surface thus became irregular. Many splits developed in the nail plate and these would give rise to white patches due to filling with air. Splitting into layers at the tip was frequent and occasionally onycholysis was noted (Calnan, 1958).

Artificial finger nails. If not made in such a way as to allow free flow of air over the nail surface, they may have an effect similar to that of the nail dressing. Severe damage can be caused, as seen in Fig. 126 where artificial finger nails had been worn to mask bitten nails (see Rein and Rogin, 1950).

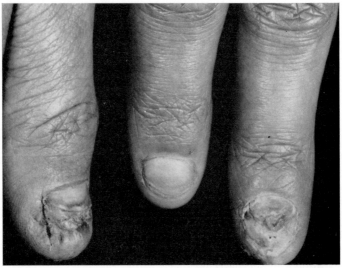

Fig. 126 Damage caused by wearing artificial nails to mask bitten nails

Artificial finger nails made from dental acrylic. When used to improve or strengthen the nails dental acrylic has to be made in situ on the nail. The liquid monomer and the powder polymer are mixed without heat and set to produce a very satisfactory 'nail' after it has been pared down by the operator. Unfortunately the liquid monomer is a potent sensitiser and patients soon get into trouble when the nails are touched up and fresh liquid has to be applied. Several types of change may occur ranging from local sepsis to onycholysis and more definite damage to the existing nail plate. Damage of this nature was recorded in the USA in 1957 but only recently has it been encountered in this country (Fisher *et al.*, 1957).

Damage caused by a base coat. Onycholysis was the principal damage caused to the nails by another nail cosmetic some years ago. This was a base coat used to improve the lasting properties of nail varnish. The material contained phenol and the damage probably resulted from the penetration of phenol through the nail plate causing irritation of the nail bed (Dobes and Nippert, 1944; Laymon and Rusten, 1949; Mitchell, 1949).

Nail hardeners containing free formalin. Onycholysis has been seen on several occasions apparently caused by the use of nail hardeners containing formaldehyde. The condition is usually limited to the tips of the nails but involves several nails. In most cases the hardener has been used more often than recommended by the manufacturers, but this is not always so. These patients have been seen in the UK and Lazar (1966) has reported the condition from the USA.

Excessive manicure, including chemical or mechanical removal of the cuticle, can distort the nail in various ways.

Damage Caused by Footwear

Ingrowing toe nails. Although the aetiology of ingrowing toe nails is disputed there seems no doubt that trauma is the major factor in their causation. In the first place unsatisfactory footwear leads to deformities of the feet then incorrect cutting of the toe nails produces spicules of nail which inflict damage to the lateral nail folds. The great toe nails are most often affected and these suffer the greatest damage during locomotion. Hyper-hidrosis is an aggravating factor.

In the early stages there is discomfort and slight local sepsis (Fig. 127) but as the condition progresses granulation tissue forms in the lateral nail fold, the infection becomes more severe and pain

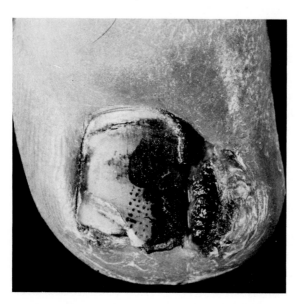

Fig. 127   Ingrowing toe nails

more intense.   The majority of cases are produced by spicules of nail penetrating the lateral nail fold.   In time, the spicule separates to a large extent from the main part of the nail and, being embedded in the soft tissues of the lateral nail fold, acts as a foreign body.   Some cases are due to over-curvature of the nail when increasing pressure results in damage to the nail fold.   A few cases develop during the treatment of fungous infection of the finger nail with griseofulvin.   The toe nails which are also diseased have become shrunken and the nail bed is also reduced in size. When treatment with griseofulvin is begun the condition of the toe nails improves to some extent, sufficiently to produce a nail which is wider than can be accommodated by the shrunken nail bed.

Many treatments for this condition have been recommended. Lloyd-Davies and Brill (1963) have shown that conservative treatment is to be recommended in most cases. They say that the patient must be instructed in foot care and sensible shoes must be worn. The nails should be cut at right angles to their long axis leaving well-defined corners. Treatment consists of soaking the feet in warm water twice daily followed by careful drying and the application of a foot powder. Caking of the powder must be avoided. A small quantity of cotton wool is then introduced gently under the corners of the nail, the patient being shown how to do this. Granulation tissue is cauterized with silver nitrate in the out-patient department. It is essential, however, that any spicule which has penetrated the nail fold be removed or continuing infection will result. This may require careful dissection to locate and remove the spicule.

With this method of treatment, cure is usually obtained in about six weeks. Operation is reserved for patients who fail to respond to conservative measures, for patients who have had the condition for a long time and demand operation, or when there is cellulitis or severe pain.

Two types of operation are recommended. The first consists of excision of granulation tissue and the lateral nail folds. The second consists of avulsion of the nail and excision of the granulation tissue and nail folds. If repeated avulsion leads to the nail being surrounded by a wall of soft tissue, ablation of the nail bed will be required.

The time-honoured partial removal of the nail is shown to be an unsatisfactory method of treatment.

Very occasionally finger or thumb nails become ingrowing. In these cases there may be no apparent trauma. Management is similar to that for toe nails.

Excess curvature in the long axis of the nail also usually affects the great toe nails. Although it may produce an ingrowing nail, sometimes it causes great discomfort from partial strangulation of the soft tissues of the distal phalanx without breaking the

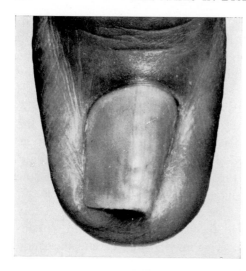

Fig. 128 Excess curvature of thumb nail. The other thumb showed the same change some months later. No cause could be found

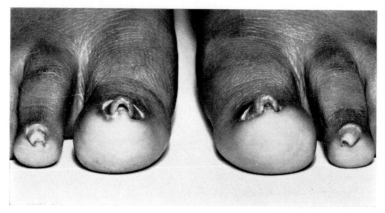

Fig. 129 Overcurvature of toe nails

epidermis. Cornelius and Shelley (1968) call this type of injury the *pincer nail syndrome*. Treatment should consist of removal of the nail plate.

Excess curvature may also be found occasionally in psoriasis and on other occasions without apparent cause. The condition may affect finger (especially thumb (Fig. 128)) or toe nails and several may be involved. Some will come to look like claws (Fig. 129).

Onychogryphosis and hypertrophied nails. In this group of disorders trauma is only one factor in its causation and some cases are probably developmental. The fact that trauma can produce hypertrophy of a nail was well illustrated by one patient with hypertrophy of a finger nail (Fig. 130). She could accurately date the commencement of the enlargement to a single injury some years previously. Onychogryphosis was once known as ostler's nail because some cases could be traced to injury caused by a horse trampling on the foot of the ostler whilst shoeing the horse.

Onychogryphosis usually affects the great toe nail but others may also be involved; the nails become thick and curved and are extremely hard to cut so that they are left untrimmed by the patient (Fig. 131). The longer they grow the greater the trauma inflicted by footwear so that the damage is progressive.

Nail hypertrophy implies thickening and increase in length whilst onychographosis implies curvature also so that the nail resembles a ram's horn. Other causes of nail hypertrophy are given on p. 20.

Treatment is difficult and can be either radical or palliative. In elderly subjects palliative treatment is preferred and consists of regular paring of the affected nails. This will usually be carried out by a chiropodist using nail clippers and file or a mechanical burr. Not infrequently the nail is invaded by granulation tissue from the nail bed and cutting into this will cause pain and haemorrhage. In younger persons the nail may be removed from time to time and allowed to regrow. The process is repeated when necessary or the nail may be permanently removed by destruction of the matrix. The latter procedure does however produce a rather unstable toe and the less destructive measure is often preferred even though it needs to be repeated occasionally.

Shedding of the toe nails. Even quite minor injury such as the wearing for a few hours of shoes which are too short may

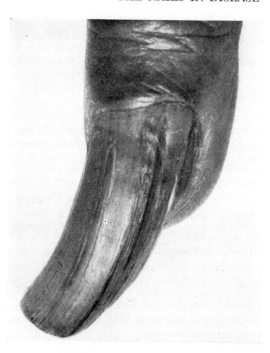

Fig. 130 Hypertrophic fingernail following trauma

Fig. 131
Onychogryphosis

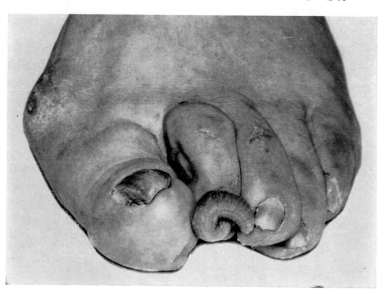

result in the formation of a subungual haematoma and this may progress to the loss of the nail some weeks later. The nail will of course be replaced in time. The great toe nails may be shed periodically in some persons, for example footballers, as a result of repeated minor injuries even in the absence of a haematoma.

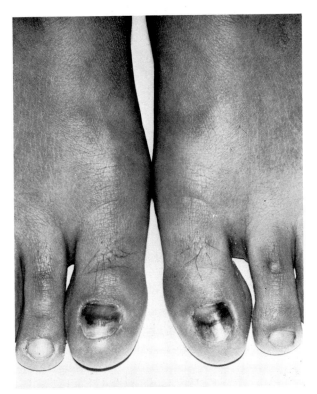

Fig. 132   Subungual haemorrhage of both great toes in patient
wearing platform shoes

The condition is probably restricted to persons with some underlying instability. Oliver (1927) described the condition in three members of a family. At times, anatomical features such as an unusually long great toe may contribute to the cause. No treatment is needed but the probable cause should be explained to the patient.

Many cases of subungual haematoma of one or both great toe nails with or without actual nail loss have recently been encountered in patients wearing platform shoes (Figs. 132 and 133). This was first noted by Almeyda (1973). The platform shoe is too rigid and during walking causes repeated minor trauma to the nail. A change to the peep-type of platform shoe should prevent recurrence.

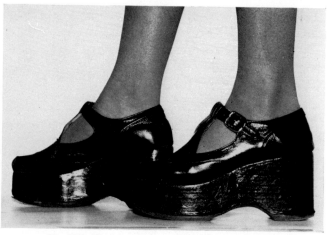

Fig. 133   Platform shoes (same patient as *Fig. 132*)

Familial periodic shedding is discussed on p. 176.

Worn down toe nails. Occasionally patients complain that some of their toe nails do not grow and it is apparent that they are being worn down by constant rubbing against the shoe. The condition is harmless and an explanation is all that is required for treatment.

References

Almeyda, J (1973) Platform nails (letter) *Brit. med. J.* **1** 176
Brodkin, R H and Bleiberg, J (1975) Cutaneous microwave injury. *Acta. Dermatoven* **53** 50
Calnan, C D (1958) Onychia from synthetic nail coverings. *Trans. St. John's Hosp. Derm. Soc. London* **41** 66
Calnan, C D (1967) Reactions to artificial colouring materials. *J. Soc. Cosmetic Chem.* **18** 215

Cohen, B H, Lewis, L A and Resnik, S S (1975) Nutcracker's nails. *Cutis.* **16** 141

Combes, F C and Scott, M J (1951) Onychotillomania. *Arch. Derm.* **63** 778

Cornelius, C and Shelley, W B (1968) Pincer nail syndrome. *Arch. Surg.* **96** 321

Dobes, W L and Nippert, P H (1944) Contact eczema due to nail polish. *Arch. Derm.* **49** 183

Farrington, G H (1964) Subungual haematoma—An evaluation of treatment. *Brit. med. J.* **1** 742

Fisher, A A, Franks, A and Glick, H (1957) Allergic sensitization of the skin and nails to acrylic plastic nails. *Journal of Allergy* **28** 84

Johnson, R K (1971) Nailplasty. *Plast. Reconstr. Surg.* **47** 275

Laymon, C W and Rusten, E M (1949) Disturbances of the nails due to base coats. *Minn. Med.* **31** 1218

Lazer, P (1966) Reactions to nail hardeners. *Arch. Derm.* **94** 446

Lloyd-Davies, R W and Brill, G G (1963) The aetiology and outpatient management of ingrowing toe nails. *Brit. J. Surg.* **50** 592

Macaulay, W L (1966) Transverse ridging of the thumb nails. *Arch. Derm.* **93** 421

Mitchell, J H (1949) Nail changes following the use of 'base coats'. *Med. Clins. N. Am.* **33** 95

Oliver, W J (1927) Recurrent onychoptosis occurring as a family disorder. *Brit. J. Derm.* **39** 297

Rein, C R and Rogin, J R (1950) Allergic eczematous reactions of the nail bed due to 'undercoats.' *Arch. Derm.* **61** 971

Samman, P D (1961) Onychia due to synthetic nail coverings. Experimental studies. *Trans. St. John's Hosp. Derm. Soc. London* **46** 68

Samman, P D (1963) A traumatic nail dystrophy produced by a habit tic. *Arch. Derm.* **88** 895

Samman, P D (1977) Nail disorders caused by external influences. *J. Soc. Cosmet. Chem.* **28** 351

Stone, O J and Mullins, J F (1963) The distal course of nail matrix haemorrhage. *Arch. Derm.* **88** 186

Chapter 11

Tumours Producing Nail Disorders

BENIGN TUMOURS

Warts

By far the commonest tumour to develop near the nail is the wart. When growing below the nail plate it often penetrates deeply like a plantar wart, but around the nail it resembles more

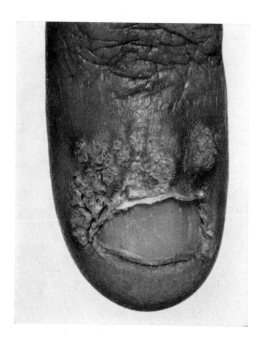

Fig. 134 Periungual warts

closely the common wart of other parts of the dorsum of the hand. Not infrequently it involves the whole of the nail fold. It is a frequent complication of nail biting (Fig. 134). The nail plate itself is only occasionally affected by the warts. It may be displaced upwards by warts under the nails and at times becomes irregular from the presence of periungual warts. Most of the damage to the nail is due to the associated nail biting. The patients almost invariably report for treatment of the warts and not for abnormalities of the nail.

It is often said that treatment of warts near the nail is difficult but generally they respond as well to conventional methods as do most multiple warts. Treatment with the electrocautery or diathermy under local anaesthesia is the method of choice for adults but in young children the author prefers to use a combination of monochloracetic acid and 40% salicylic acid plaster. This method of treatment was detailed by Halpern and Lane (1953). A saturated solution of monochloracetic acid is applied to the wart by a wisp of cotton wool around the end of an orange stick. When dry it is covered with 40% salicylic acid plaster cut to the size of the wart and this is held in place by two or three layers of zinc oxide adhesive tape. The patient is instructed to remove the plasters after three days and to apply a light dressing if necessary. The patient is seen again after 7–14 days when many of the warts may be picked out or the treatment repeated if necessary. At the first visit the acid should be applied rather sparingly, as keratin will take up a considerable quantity if allowed to do so. A too liberal application will result in pus formation and pain but no permanent damage to the nail fold which shows remarkable powers of regeneration. It is usually unnecessary to pare down the wart before the acid is applied. Unlike trichloracetic acid, monochloracetic acid does not whiten the skin when applied.

For warts below the nail it is necessary to cut away the overlying nail before treatment is started. Again electrocautery or diathermy is often the method of choice but the author has found that a number of these will respond to 3% formalin. The finger tip is held in the formalin solution for 10–15 minutes daily for 14–21 days. If the wart does not harden and die within this time it is unwise to continue as formalin dermatitis may develop.

Periungual Fibroma

Fibromata growing from the nail fold are frequent stigmata of adenoma sebaceum but are at times seen without other evidence of this disorder (Fig. 135). They cause little real disability but give rise to some inconvenience and at times may be the cause of a depression forming on the nail plate.

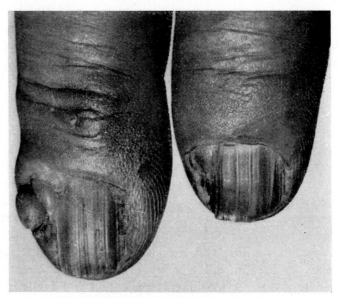

Fig. 135 Periungual fibromata

The diagnosis is usually obvious and treatment is by excision if requested. Histologically they may show vascular lakes near the tip (Pardo-Castello and Pardo, 1960).

Garlic Clove Fibroma

Under this heading, Steel (1965) described a small tumour growing away from the nail bed and projecting from the cuticle over the finger or toe. It is loosely attached by a pedicle. The tumour is either a benign epitheliomatous polyp or an irritation fibroma of the nail bed. Histological examination shows that it is covered, except at its base, by a layer of stratified squamous epithelium. The core is composed of interlacing bundles of dense collagenous tissue with capillary channels. Treatment is by excision. Undeutsch and Shrieferstein (1974) describe a similar condition under the heading garlic corm fibroma.

A small filamentous tumour growing below the nail and extending the whole length of the nail plate has been seen by the author on a number of occasions. It presents at the tip of the digit below the nail and can be traced under the nail plate to the cuticle. The nail may be slightly ridged over it. The nosology of this tumour has not yet been determined but it may be a subungual fibroma. It normally causes no trouble so that treatment is not required. It pares down painlessly when the nail is cut.

Subungual Exostosis

This is not very uncommon and is most often seen on the great toes. It presents as a firm swelling below the nail near the tip and in time will displace the nail (Fig. 136). It is often mis-

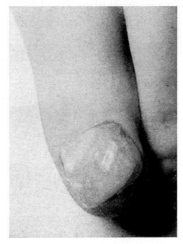

Fig. 136   Subungual exostosis

taken for a wart. X-ray will establish the diagnosis in every case (Fig. 137) (Evison, 1966). It is not a true exostosis but an outgrowth of normal bone. Treatment is by excision with strict aseptic precautions because the outgrowth from the distal phalanx must be cut away.

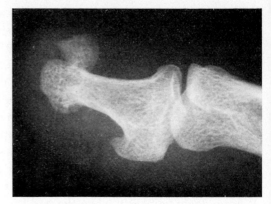

Fig. 137 Same as *Fig. 136*—
X-ray

Mucous Cyst

This is not a true tumour but a collagenous degeneration of the extensor tendon presenting as a tumour; it has often in the past been designated a synovial cyst. The condition almost always forms on the dorsum of the distal phalanx between the distal interphalangeal joint and the base of the nail. It is usually quite

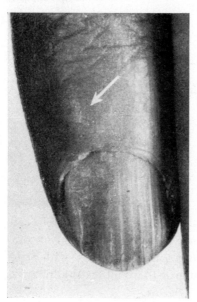

Fig. 138 Mucous cyst—small lesion arrowed. The ridging on the nail is incidental

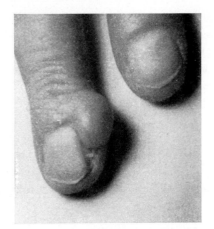

Fig. 139 Mucous cyst—large lesion

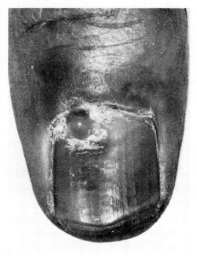

(a)

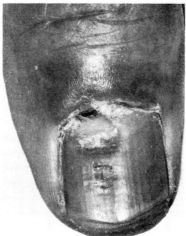

(b)

Fig. 140 (a) and (b) Fluid escaping
    from a mucous cyst

small (Fig. 138), but occasionally quite large (Fig. 139). It frequently deforms the nail by producing a depression, 1–2 mm across, throughout the length of the nail. A small quantity of the contents of the cyst escapes down the groove below the cuticle from time to time (Fig. 140). The lesion often accompanies osteoarthritis of the adjacent interphalangeal joint.

Except for the nail deformity, the condition is harmless but if it is deforming the nail or is unsightly because of its size it should be excised (Arner *et al.*, 1956) or a few drops of a depot steroid (e.g. methyl prednisolone) may be injected. No treatment is perfect and the condition may relapse even after excision.

Glomus Tumour

This is a rare tumour which may develop in the corium of the nail bed giving rise to great pain. The pain may be spontaneous or occur with pressure. The lesion is minute but can usually be seen through the nail plate as a bluish discoloration. It arises from hypertrophy of a glomus body. Treatment should consist of total excision with full aseptic precautions. If not completely removed, recurrence is probable.

Pigmented Naevus

In white persons a longitudinal band of pigment in the nail plate may be due to a junctional naevus in the nail matrix (Harvey, 1960) (Fig. 141). The effect is due to a spill of pigment into the nail plate. It may start at any age, but once it begins it tends to persist indefinitely. These lesions have been known to become malignant. For lesions on the toe nails and the less important finger nails it is wise therefore to recommend removal of the nail followed by excision of the affected area of the matrix and suture of the cut edges. This procedure will leave a ridge or even a permanent split in the nail when it regrows, so that for the thumb and index finger a policy of wait and watch is justified.

Pigment streaks in the nails in coloured people are much more common and are due to minor trauma (p. 128).

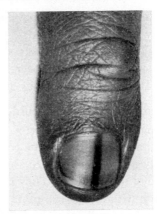

Fig. 141 Pigment band probably due to a junctional naevus

Enchondroma

This tumour is very rarely encountered in the distal phalanx when it may present either as chronic paronychia (Shelley and Ralston, 1964) or with greater distortion of the nail (Yaffee, 1965). X-ray will show a radiolucent defect with expansion of the distal phalanx. Treatment is by removal of the chondroid tissue and by filling the cavity so formed with a bone graft if necessary. The condition must be distinguished from an epithelioma or a malignant melanoma which may present in the same way.

Keratoacanthoma

This tumour is relatively common on the face and diagnosis is easily established but when occurring below the nail is uncommon and quite unlike the classical lesion (Lamp, 1964). It presents as redness and swelling of the tips of the digit with increasing pain. For a few weeks progress is rapid and it may mimic chronic paronychia. Part of the nail separates from the nail bed and a crusted nodule appears at the edge. X-ray shows extensive destruction of the distal phalanx. Histology is the same as in the classical lesion and may easily be mistaken for an epithelioma. Treatment is by excision after removal of the overlying nail, but partial amputation is not required.

Pyogenic Granuloma

A classical pyogenic granuloma near the nail is somewhat rare but if it occurs it should be removed with curette and cautery.

As a malignant melanoma may present in this way, this possibility must be considered.

Excess granulation tissue simulating a pyogenic granuloma is much more common, especially in relation to an ingrowing toe nail. It should be treated as described under that heading.

Subungual Epidermoid Inclusions

These have been described by Lewin (1969) as bulbous proliferations of the tips of the rete ridges below the nail. They are usually microscopic in size and found only on histological examination of the nail bed. They occur especially with finger clubbing but also without this symptom. They may be the result of trauma. Very occasionally they become large enough to cause symptoms and must therefore be considered in the differential diagnosis of nail bed swellings.

MALIGNANT TUMOURS

Epithelioma

Epithelioma of the nail bed is a rare form of malignancy (Gelmann, 1963). It is most likely to present as a chronic paronychia with increasing pain (Fig. 142), but may present as an outgrowth from below the edge of the nail. It may also begin as a pyogenic granuloma (Driban and Lacagnata, 1975). Biopsy is

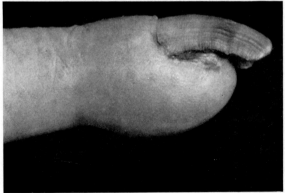

Fig. 142 Epithelioma of nail bed presenting as chronic paronychia

essential to establish the diagnosis. Treatment should be partial amputation of the digit. The prognosis is good.

Bowen's disease of the nail bed is also rare but should be suspected in any case of gradual destruction of a single nail in the absence of a fungal infection. The condition is liable to progress to an invasive carcinoma. Treatment may be partial amputation of the digit but Moh's chemosurgical technique will give a better cosmetic result (Mikhail, 1974).

Secondary carcinoma may occasionally settle in the bone of the distal phalanx giving rise to a painful swelling. X-ray will usually establish the diagnosis, if a primary site is known, but a biopsy may be required.

Malignant Melanoma

This also is a rare tumour below the nail but one in which early diagnosis is essential. It may present in various ways. First

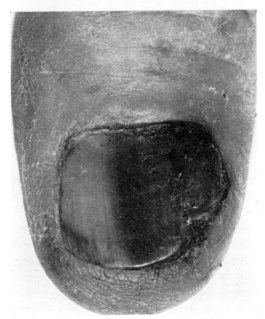

Fig. 143 Malignant melanoma developing from a junctional naevus

as a chronic paronychia when the appearance of pigment on the surface of the digit spreading out from below the nail should give rise to suspicion. It may develop from a junctional naevus (p. 156) and in that case the pigment band on the nail will become wider (Fig. 143) and granulation tissue may develop at the nail edge. Granulation tissue resembling a pyogenic granuloma without the added pigment band in the nail is another presentation. It may also present as a warty thickening of the nail bed with shedding of

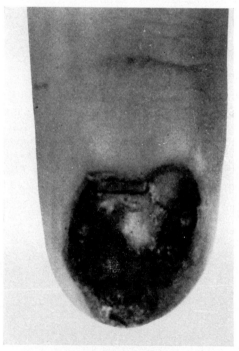

Fig. 144 Malignant melanoma

the nail (Fig. 144). In any case of doubt a biopsy should be made after a tourniquet has been placed round the finger, and a frozen section examined. If the diagnosis is confirmed, immediate amputation of the digit should be undertaken and the regional glands should be removed at a later date if necessary.

Prognosis is good if diagnosis is established early and treatment instituted without delay, unfortunately diagnosis may at times be much delayed (Leppard *et al.*, 1974).

References

Arner, O, Lindholm, A and Romanus, R (1956) Mucous cysts of the fingers. *Acta. Chir. Scand.* **3** 314

Driban, N E and Lacagnata, J T (1975) Subungual Squamous Cell Carcinoma. *Dermatologica* **150** 186

Evision G (1966) Subungual exostosis. *Brit. J. Radiol* **39** 451

Gelmann, S B (1963) Primary carcinoma of the nail bed. *N. Y. St. J. Med.* **63** 2408

Halpern, L K and Lane, C W (1953) Treatment of periungual warts. *Missouri Med.* **50** 765

Harvey, K M (1960) Pigmented naevus of nail. *Lancet* **ii** 848

Lamp, J C, Graham, J H, Urbach, F and Burgoon, F. Jr. (1964) Keratoacanthoma of the subungual region. *J. Bone Jt. Surg.* **46A** 1721

Leppard, B, Sanderson, K V and Behan F (1974) Subungual malignant melanoma: difficulty in diagnosis. *Brit. med. J.* **1** 310

Lewin, K (1969) Subungual epidermoid inclusions. *Brit. J. Derm.* **81** 671

Mikhail, G R (1974) Bowen's disease and squamous cell carcinoma of the nail bed. *Arch. Derm.* **110** 267

Pardo-Castello, V and Pardo, O A (1960) Diseases of the nails. *3rd Ed., p.* **90** *C. C. Thomas, Springfield, Illinois*

Shelley, W B and Ralston, E I (1964) Paronychia due to enchondroma. *Arch. Derm.* **90** 412

Steel, H H (1965) Garlic clove fibroma. *J. Am. med. Ass.* **191** 1082

Undeutsch, W and Shrieferstein, G (1974) Garlic corm fibroma. *Dermatologica* **149** 110

Yaffee, M S (1965) Peculiar nail dystrophy caused by an enchondroma. *Arch. Derm.* **91** 361

Chapter 12

Developmental Anomalies

Although all rather uncommon developmental anomalies of the nails form an interesting group of disorders, there are a few well recognized congenital abnormalities and a few other conditions which appear to be developmental but the genetic cause has not yet been firmly established.

Pachyonychia Congenita

The term appears first to have been used by Jadassohn and Lewandowski (1906) to describe a case. Their case had dystrophic nails, palmar and plantar hyperkeratosis, hyperhidrosis and blistering of the feet during the summer months, excess sweating of the nose and leukokeratosis of the tongue. There have been numerous reports in the literature describing individual cases of

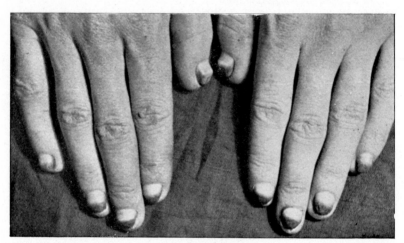

Fig. 145 Pachyonychia congenita. (*Reproduced from Proceedings of the Royal Society of Medicine by permission of the Editors*)

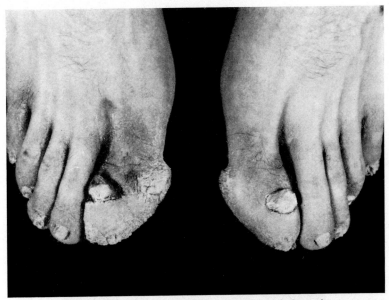

Fig. 146 Pachyonychia congenita with hyperkeratotic formations

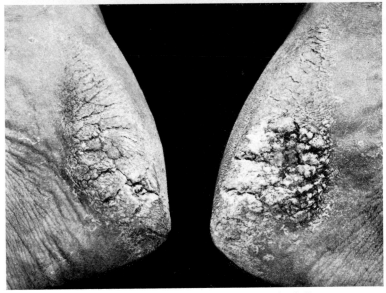

Fig. 147 Pachyonychia congenita—hyperkeratosis of elbows

families which show several of these features and others in which the symptomatology is rather different. It is probable that there are a number of different syndromes involved. All are inherited as an autosomal dominant but it is uncertain if one or more genes is involved. Kumer and Loos (1935) suggest that there are three main variants. It is suggested that there are probably four different syndromes as described below.

Type 1. This is probably the most common and corresponds largely to the original type of Jadassohn and Lewandowski. The nails are usually normal at birth but within the first year of life

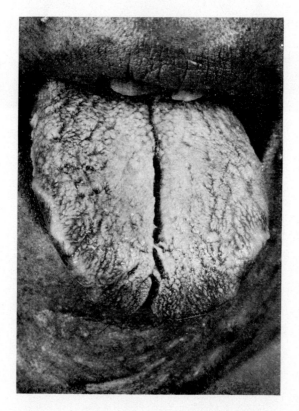

Fig. 148 Pachyonychia congenita—tongue showing
leukokeratosis

and often in the first few days they become discoloured and
thicken progressively from base to tip so that they appear wedge
shaped (Fig. 145). This change is seen better on the fingers than
the toe nails which are more uniformally thickened. In addition
to the nail changes there are characteristically palmar and
plantar hyperkeratoses (Fig. 146) and warty lesions on knees,

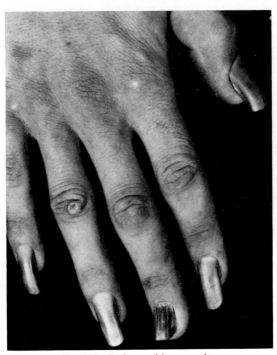

Fig. 149   Pachyonychia congenita

elbows, (Fig. 147) buttocks, legs, ankles and in the popliteal
region. Bullae appear on the feet in association with hyperhidrosis and may be crippling. In the mouth especially on the
tongue (Fig. 148) there may be dyskeratosis. In some cases corneal
dyskeratosis has been described but has not been seen by the
author.

Type 2. In this type the nail thickening is more uniform and
some of the nails may be infected with candida (Fig. 149). There

is also chronic candidiasis in the mouth and this suggests some immune defect. Keratoses are much less severe than in type 1. Patients with chronic oral candidiasis and pachyonycyhia congenita were shown at the Royal Society of Medicine by Higgs (1973) and Forman and Wells (1975).

Type 3. This is perhaps the most interesting group and is really very different from the others. Affected children have erupted teeth at birth. Soderquist and Reed (1968) describe such a family. All affected members had two to six teeth at birth. The premature teeth are usually soft and quickly shed but as they normally replace the corresponding milk teeth the children are partially edentulous until the permanent teeth erupt. In this type hyperkeratoses are relatively insignificant and the nail thickening is much less severe than in types 1 and 2. As noted by Shrank (1966) Soderquist and Reed (1968) adults in these families may have multiple epidermal cysts and there may be other congenital anomalies. Vineyard and Scott (1961) describe the association of sebocystomatosis and pachyonychia congenita and the author has seen such a case in this group. There may also be abnormalities of the hair. It has been variously reported as dry, lustreless and kinky (Soderquist and Reed, 1968); short and straight and with eye brows which stand straight out (Boxley, 1971).

Type 4. The characteristic feature in this group is a widespread macular pigmentation affecting especially the neck and axillae. Nail changes and keratoses are of moderate severity.

In addition to the family groups, isolated cases are encountered in which abnormalities are confined to the nails. They should not be called pachyonychia congenita in the absence of other stigmata or a clear cut family history.

Treatment of the whole group is far from satisfactory. The nails should be kept well trimmed and this requires the use of nail clippers. At times the removal of nail and matrix will be required. Some regrowth from the nail bed should be expected. Hyperkeratotic formations may be helped by the use of salicylic acid or urea ointments. Vitamin A in high dosage has helped some patients, in respect both of keratoses and leukokeratosis.

The Nail Patella Syndrome

This is a curious condition affecting both mesodermal and ectodermal structures. The principal abnormalities consist of nail changes, small or absent patellae, abnormalities of elbow joints, iliac horns and in a minority of cases renal changes. It is inherited as an autosomal dominant with linkage between the locus controlling the gene and that of the ABO blood groups (Renwick and Lawler, 1955).

The typical case shows nails which are grossly defective, $\frac{1}{3}$ to $\frac{1}{2}$ the normal size and never reaching the finger tip making it very difficult to pick up small objects. The change is seen more often in women than men. In some cases the entire thumb nail is missing (Fig. 150) or it may be represented by a fringe of hard keratin

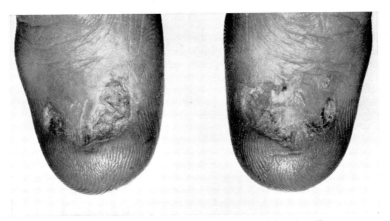

Fig. 150 Nail patella syndrome—total loss of thumb nails

in the nail fold. Although there is scarring it is obvious that the nail bed is present. In the least affected cases only the ulnar half of each thumb nail is missing (Fig. 151) whilst other nails are normal. Levan (1961) described a case of this type and gave a useful bibliography. In every case the thumb nails are most

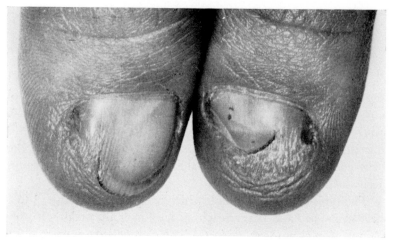

Fig. 151 Nail-patella syndrome—loss of ulnar half of thumb nails

affected and changes if present in other nails diminish progressively from index to little finger. A change often seen in the less severely affected nails is a split near the centre dividing the nail and each half may be spoon shaped. A V-shaped half moon is also rather characteristic and is the only abnormality seen on some nails (Fig. 152).

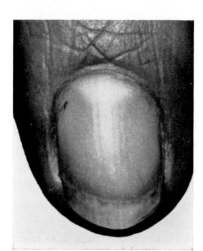

Fig. 152 Nail-patella syndrome—
V-shaped half moon

The abnormality of the patella consists of reduction in size or actual absence. Although the knee appears unstable this abnormality in fact causes very little inconvenience.

The elbow joints usually show an obvious deformity. The carrying angle is increased and there is limited supination and incomplete extension of the elbow. In some cases an abnormality is visible only on X-ray. This shows a disorganised joint in which a poorly formed and subluxated head of the radius is articulated with a small underdeveloped capitellum. These changes also cause little inconvenience.

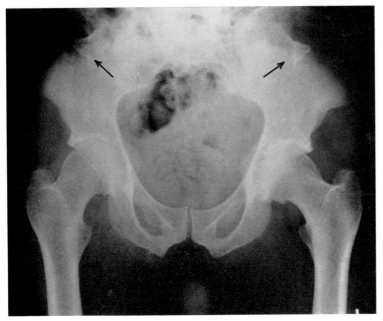

Fig. 153 Nail patella syndrome—X-ray pelvis showing iliac spines (arrowed)

Iliac horns when large, may be palpated but usually are only seen on X-ray (Fig. 153). They arise from the centre of the external aspect of the ilium and project in a posterolateral direction.

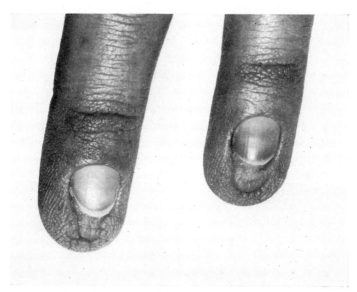

Fig. 154 Congenital ectodermal defect (hidrotic type): Fingers showing
failure of nails to grow to full length and mammilation of finger tips

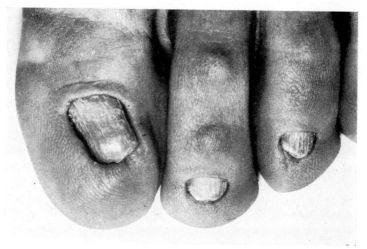

Fig. 155 Congenital ectodermal defect (hidrotic type): toe nails showing
thickening and ridging

The renal changes clinically are those of chronic glomerulo-nephritis with persistent albuminuria and casts of all types and occasional red blood cells in the urine. Renal function may be diminished (Hawkins and Smith, 1950). Although the other changes are usually present in all affected individuals the renal changes are inconstant and are the only serious feature of the syndrome. Goodman and Cuppage (1967) and Ben Bassat *et al.* (1971) have examined the kidney under the electronmicroscope and showed that the changes include thickening and wrinkling of the glomerular basement membrane.

Anonychia

Apart from the nail patella syndrome anonychia (absence of the nail from birth) is encountered very rarely. Littman and Levin (1964) described a girl with seven nails missing and her brother was similarly affected. They considered the condition to be an autosomal recessive genetic defect. In anonychia with ectrodactyly (Lees *et al.*, 1957) several nails may be missing and there are often bizarre associated defects of the digits. This is an autosomal dominant condition. Feinmesser and Zelig (1961) described two children of a sibship of five with rudimentary nails and an associated congenital deafness. Verbov (1975) described a case with anonychia, bizarre flexural pigmentation, hypo-hidrosis and dry palmar and plantar skin which partly destroyed the normal skin markings. Other members of the family were similarly affected with autosomal dominant inheritance.

Bart (1971) gives details of a family showing a unique com-bination of localised absence of the skin, blistering of skin and mucous membranes and nail abnormalities. The nail defor-mities consist of congenital absence, or subsequent loss and other changes. He refers to an earlier description of the family in which the blistering was likened to epidermolysis bullosa. The condition showed an autosomal dominant mode of inheritance.

Congenital Ectodermal Defect

There are a number of different syndromes described under

this heading the main division being into anhidrotic and hidrotic types. In the *anhidrotic type* nail changes are an insignificant feature but they may be thin, brittle and ridged.

Hidrotic type. This condition is inherited as an autosomal dominant and many of the recorded cases can be traced to a small region in France. Clouston (1929) described a large number of cases from French speaking Canada. The nails were involved in every case and hair in 50% of cases.

Various nail changes have been described. The most characteristic seen in several patients by the author is a nail which grows

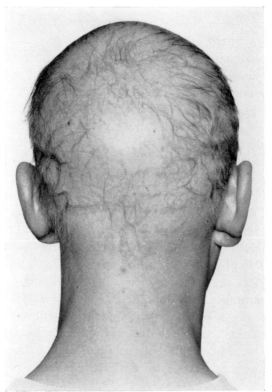

Fig. 156 Congenital ectodermal defect (hidrotic type): same patient as in *Figs. 154* and *155* showing associated alopecia

slowly and never reaches the finger tip. Surrounding the nail and on the finger tip including the nail bed left exposed by the failure of the nail to reach the tip is a curious mammilation (Fig. 154). This is seen on all fingers. Onycholysis is the principal feature in other cases and this may be accompanied by subungual sepsis and malodour. Toe nails are more often thickened (Fig. 155) and the mammilation less obvious. Pachyonychial changes are present sometimes. Other nail changes have been described but it is not clear from the literature that they refer to the hidrotic type and there is undoubted confusion between this condition and the nail patella syndrome.

Alopecia (Fig. 156) seen in half the cases may involve the scalp alone or be universal. There are often hyperkeratotic formations on the soles and elsewhere.

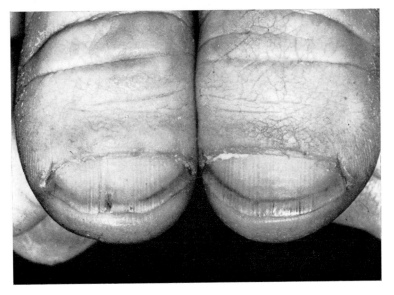

Fig. 157 Nail en raquette

Dyskeratosis congenita. Various nail abnormalities have been recorded in this very rare disorder (Cole *et al.*, 1930).

Racket Nail

(nail en raquette)

This is in fact a congenital abnormality of the thumb (*le pouce en raquette*) with the nail conforming to the altered shape of the thumb. It is very much more common than the other conditions described here. It is inherited as an autosomal dominant but is rather more common in women than men. Basset (1962) says twice as common and Ronchese (1973) three times as common. It may affect one or both thumbs. The distal phalanx is shorter and wider than usual and the nail is also short and wide and the lateral curvature is lost (Fig. 157). Of 63 cases investigated by Ronchese (1951) 31 gave a family history.

Basset (1962) distinguished this from two similar conditions. In one the racket shape affects all fingers and in the other the thumb nails are short but without the corresponding shortening of the distal phalanges.

Supernumerary Digits

These are usually provided with a normal nail but when rudimentary there may either be no sign of the nail or nail matrix or the tip is provided with a vestigial nail (Fig. 158).

Additional nails

Very occasionally instead of one nail there are two nails on a digit, usually both rather abnormal (Fig. 159).

Kikuchi *et al.* (1974) describe a clinical entity which they call *congenital onychodysplasia of the index fingers* and refer to other reports of a similar nature. The condition is limited to the index fingers and the nails may be absent, small or multiple. It is non hereditary and non familial and except perhaps for the case illustrated here (Fig. 159) which may be the same condition as it affected the index finger, all cases have come from Japan.

Leukonychia Totalis

This is a rare developmental abnormality inherited as an autosomal dominant. The entire nail plate is white and the

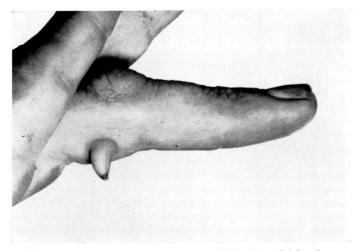

Fig. 158 Rudimentary supernumerary digit with vestigial nail

Fig. 159 Additional nail

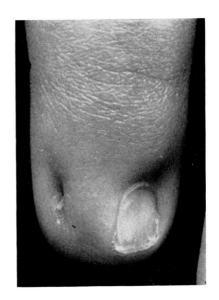

whiteness is due to changes in the nail plate itself (Plate III (*a*)).
The material of the nail is poor and it may become brittle,

broken and discoloured distally (Fig. 160). In many cases multiple epidermal cysts are also present.

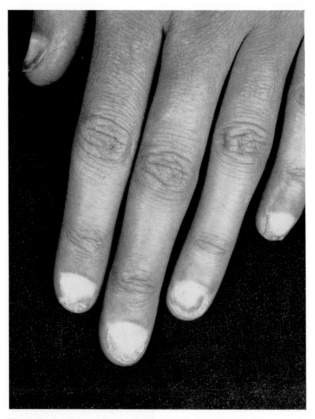

Fig. 160   Leukonychia totalis—material of nail plate is poor and
the edges have become discoloured and broken

Periodic Shedding

Another rare developmental abnormality which is inherited as an autosomal dominant. One or more nails is repeatedly shed and replaced. The new nail may be imperfect and this leads to considerable deformities (Fig. 161). The nails on various digits are shed independently so that there is seldom more than one missing at a time.

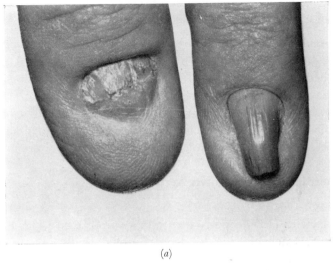

(a)

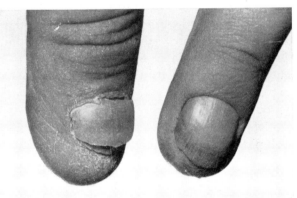

(b)

Fig. 161   Periodic shedding (a) mother (b) son

The true congenital condition must be distinguished from shedding due to other causes and in particular from trauma due to footwear.

A very curious case of nail shedding was described by Frank and Sanford (1891). Their patient shed his whole epidermis including all nails on the same day every year for 45 years. Other cases of a similar nature have been recorded.

Hereditary koilonychia has been described on p. 111. Onycholysis has been fully described on p. 20. A developmental form described as *hereditary partial onycholysis* has been described by Schulze (1966). Sparrow *et al.* (1976) recorded details of a family showing hyperpigmentation, hypohidrosis, nail dystrophy, hypoplasia of dermatoglyphics and a number of other abnormalities. The main nail change was extensive onycholysis.

Condition of Unknown Aetiology

Rough Nails (Trachyonychie)

Alkiewiez (1950) and Achten and Wanet-Rouard (1974) use the term trachyonychie to describe rough nails. Baran and Dupré (1977) elaborate and say that rough nails are suggestive of some cases of alopecia areata and use the term '*vertical striated sandpaper nails*' to describe these cases. When the vertical striations do not cover the full expanse of the nail plates the condition they say may be due to lichen planus or psoriasis.

The author has seen many cases of rough nails which are very difficult to place aetiologically and roughly divides them into the following groups:

Universal pitting with variants excess ridging and rippling

Excess ridging (not a manifestation of universal pitting) and sometimes called '20 nail dystrophy'.

Severe nail dystrophy

Regular pitting

Many cases of uniform pitting of the nails can be attributed to psoriasis (Klingmüller and Reh, 1955) or to alopecia areata (Stühmer, 1957) but when these conditions have been excluded, by personal and family history and by examination, some unexplained cases remain (Fig. 162). Several examples have been

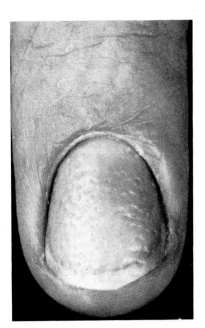

Fig. 162 Regular pitting—cause unknown

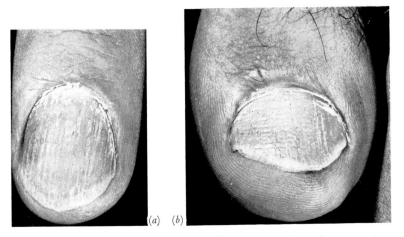

(a)   (b)

Fig. 163   (a) ridging of a finger nail   (b) rippling of a toe nail from the same patient
on the same day

seen in more than one member of a family so that some genetic
basis is probable. The pits usually appear early in life but may
become manifest years later. One or many nails are affected. The
patient can observe the change starting as pits which become
visible in the half moon area and progress forwards to involve the
whole nail. Mottling in the half moon is sometimes present. The
condition may gradually clear spontaneously but more often it is
permanent. It is apparent that there is an intermittent defect of
parts of the matrix the cause of which is as yet unknown.

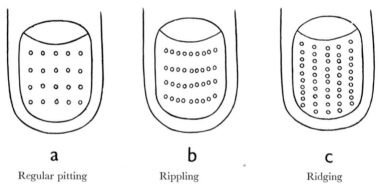

a   b   c

Regular pitting   Rippling   Ridging

Fig. 164   Diagrams to show how regular pitting could be converted to rippling
or ridging

Excess ridging and rippling

These two conditions appear at times to be variants of uniform
pitting and patients have been seen where all three abnormalities
were present at the same time on different digits (Fig. 163). The
manner in which regular pitting could produce these changes is
shown in Fig. 164 (*a*), (*b*) and (*c*). As the aetiology is obscure it is
possible that there is more than one cause and not every case will
be genetically determined. Rippling gives a very characteristic
picture likened to the ripples on the sand of the sea shore after the
tide has gone out (Fig. 165).

Excess ridging or *twenty nail dystrophy of childhood*

Hazelrigg *et al.* (1977) give this name to a condition which was
described in earlier editions of *The nails in disease* under the heading

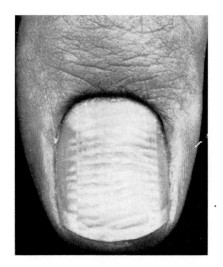

Fig. 165   Rippling

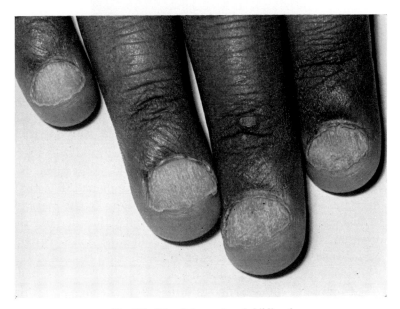

Fig. 166   20 nail dystrophy of childhood

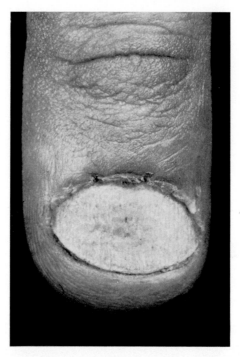

Fig. 167   Finger nail showing excess ridging

of excess ridging. Excess ridging appears to be the primary defect and in this case is not due to multiple pits running together. The child is born with normal nails but after a few months or years all nails become excessively ridged (Fig. 166). The ridging starts at the cuticle and progresses to the tip. There are so many lines close together that the nail looses its lustre and become opalescent. The end result is a rather ugly nail (Fig. 167). There are no related skin or hair abnormalities. In the majority of cases there is no family history of a similar disorder but the author has seen two cases in one family, both girls. The dystrophy is at its worst in the early stage and gradually decreases with age. As it is not encountered in adults it seems probable that eventually it clears entirely. Treatment has little effect on progress but the use of nail lacquer hides the defect.

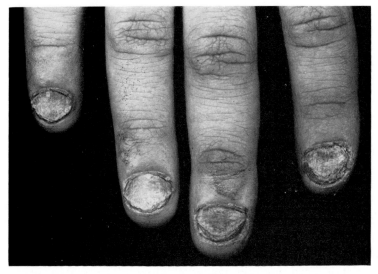

Fig. 168 Severe nail dystrophy

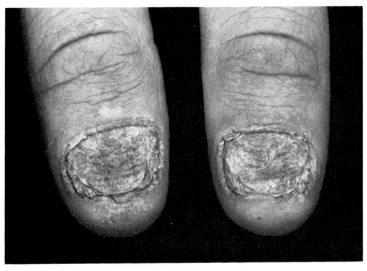

Fig. 169 Severe nail dystrophy

Severe nail dystrophy

This is another condition usually seen in childhood and affecting many nails. It has to be distinguished from psoriasis and alopecia areata affecting the nails and this may not be easy. The nails are affected in a variety of ways and all types of change may occur at the same time, one nail showing one form whilst others show another. Often some nails are completely spared. Most nails are soft and slightly discoloured. They are opalescent and lack lustre (Fig. 168 and 169). Some are thicker than normal but some are thin. Pitting or ridging may be present but is not a prominent feature. Some nails, especially thumb or great toe nails, show marked koilonychia. Although most cases are seen in young children and, as in the 20 nail dystrophy, there is a gradual improvement with age, a few cases have been adults. Injections of triamcinolone have improved the adult cases but have not been used in young children. The author usually recommends the use of a relatively mild topical steroid but it is uncertain whether this treatment really helps.

Great Toe Nail Dystrophy

Under this heading the author (Samman, 1978) has described a condition confined to one or both great toe nails. The nail changes are present at birth. The nail is dark coloured, slightly pointed but shorter than a normal nail (Fig. 170). Cross ridges may develop on its surface and a large portion of the nail may be shed from time to time. In a number of cases the condition has been entirely symptomless except for the disfigurement but in one child, after shedding of part of the nail, ingrowth into the nail bed occurred on regrowth so that the nail had to be removed surgically. The condition is probably permanent.

Macronychia and Micronychia

Nails which are larger (macro) or smaller (micro) (Fig. 171) than normal but in all other respects quite normal. The condition may affect one or more nails and be unilateral or bilateral.

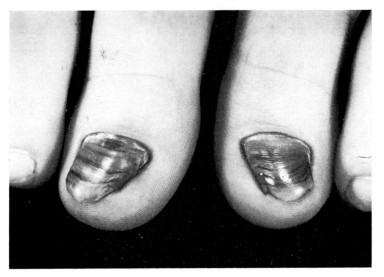

Fig. 170 Great toe nail dystrophy

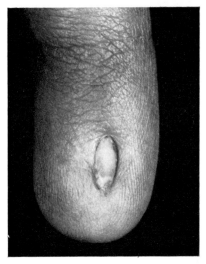

Fig. 171 Micronychia

Claw-like Little Toe Nails

These are not very uncommon. One or both little toe nails are rounded like a claw. The condition is often associated with hyperkeratotic formations on the feet or elsewhere. Much less often other toe nails show this change.

References

Achten, G and Wanet-Rouard, J (1974) Atrophie unguale et trachyonychie. *Arch. Belges Dermatol.* **30** 201

Alkiewicz, J (1950) Trachyonychie. *Ann. Dermatol. Syphiligr.* **10** 136

Baran, R and Dupré, A (1977) Vertical striated sandpaper nails (letter) *Arch. Derm.* **113** 1613

Bart, B J (1971) Congenital localised absence of skin, blistering and nail abnormalities, a new syndrome. Birth defects: original article series **7** 118

Basset, M R H (1962) Trois formes génotypiques d'ongles courts: le pouce en raquette, les doigts en raquette, les ongles courts simples. *Bull. Soc. fr. Derm. Syph.* **69** 15

Ben-Bassat, M, Cohen, L and Rosenfeld, J (1971) The glomerular basement membrane in the nail patella syndrome. *Arch. Path.* **92** 350

Besser, F S (1971) Pachyonychia congenita with epidermal cysts and teeth at birth: 4th generation. *Brit. J. Derm.* **84** 95

Boxley, J D (1971) Pachyonychia congenita and multiple epidermal hamatomata. *Brit. J. Derm.* **85** 298

Clouston, H R (1929) A Hereditary Ectodermal Dystrophy. *Canad. med. Ass. J.* **21** 18

Cole, H N, Raushkolb, J E and Toomey, J (1930) Dyskeratosis congenita with Pigmentation, Dystrophia unguis and leukokeratosis oris. *Arch. Derm.* **21** 71

Feinmesser, M and Zelig, S (1961) Congenital deafness associated with onychodystrophy. *Arch. Otolar.* **74** 507

Forman, L and Wells, R S (1975) Pachyonychia congenita and chronic candidiasis of the mouth in a father and two children. *Proc. Roy. Soc. Med.* **68** 762

Frank, J and Sanford, W C (1891) A remarkable case of skin disease. *Amer. J. med. Sci.* **102** 164

Goodman R M and Cuppage, F E (1967) The nail patella syndrome. Clinical findings and ultrastructural observations in the kidney. *Arch. intern. Med.* **120** 68

Hawkins, C F and Smith, O E (1950) Renal dysplasia in a family with multiple hereditary abnormalities including iliac horns. *Lancet* **i** 803

Hazelrigg, D E Duncan, C and Jarratt, M (1977) Twenty nail dystrophy of childhood. *Arch. Derm.* **113** 75

Higgs, J M (1973) Pachyonychia congenita and chronic oral candidiasis. *Proc. Roy. Soc. Med.* **66** 628

Jadassohn, von J and Lewandowski, F (1906) Pachyonychia congenita. Keratosis disseminata circumscripta tylomata et keratosis linguae. *Ikonographia Dermatologica*

Klingmüller, G and Reh, E (1955) Nagelbrübchen und deren familiäre Haüfungen bei der Alopecia areata. *Arch. klin. exp. Derm.* **201** 574

Kumer, L and Loos, H O (1955) Uber pachyonychia congenita (typus Riehl). *Wein, klin. Wsch.* **6** 174

Lees, D H, Lawler, S D, Renwick, J H and Thoday, J M (1957) Anonychia with ectrodactyly: clinical and linkage data. *Ann. hum. Genet.* **22** 69

Levan, N E (1961) Congenital defect of thumb nails. *Arch. Derm.* **83** 938

Littman, A and Levin, S (1964) Anonychia as a Recessive Autosomal trait in man. *J. invest. Derm.* **42** 177

Murray, F A (1921) Congenital anomalies of the nails. Four cases of hereditary hypertrophy of the nail-bed associated with a history of erupted teeth at birth. *Brit. J. Derm.* **33** 409

Renwick, J H and Lawler, S D (1955) Genetical linkage between the A B O and nail patella loci. *Ann. hum. Genet.* (*Lond.*) **19** 312

Ronchese, F (1951) Peculiar nail anomalies. *Arch. Derm.* **63** 565

Ronchese, F (1973) The racket thumb-nail. *Dermatologica* **146** 199

Samman, P D (1978) Great toe nail dystrophy. *Clin & Exper. Derm.* **3** 81

Schulze, H D (1966) Hereditäre onycholysis partialis mit Skleronychie. *Derm. Wschr.* **152** 766

Shrank, A B (1966) Pachyonychia congenita (case report). *Proc. Roy. Soc. Med.* **59** 975

Soderquist, N A and Reed, W B (1968) Pachyonychia congenita with epidermal cysts and other congenital dyskeratoses. *Arch. Derm.* **97** 31

Sparrow, G P, Samman, P D and Wells, R S (1976) Hyperpigmentation and hypohidrosis. *Clin & Exper. Derm.* **1** 127

Stühmer, A (1957) Rhythmen im biologischen Gescheben bei gesunden und kranken Nägeln. *Arch. klin. exp. Derm.* **204** 1

Verbov, J (1975) Anonychia with bizarre flexural pigmentation—an autosomal dominant dermatosis *Brit. J. Derm.* **92** 469

Vineyard, W R and Scott, R A (1961) Steatocystoma multiplex with pachyonychia congenita. *Arch. Derm.* **84** 824

Appendix I

GLOSSARY OF TERMS USED IN NAIL DISEASES

Acaulosis unguis Infection of nail with *Scopulariopsis brevicaulis*

Agnail Hang nail; hard spicules at edge of nail

Anonychia Absence of the nail

Defluvium unguium Nail shedding, starting at base and extending forward

Fragilitas unguium Brittle nails

Hapalonychia Soft nails

Koilonychia Spoon-shaped nails

Leukonychia White nails

Macronychia Large but otherwise normal nails

Micronychia Small but otherwise normal nails

Onychalgia nervosa Exquisitely sensitive nails

Onychauxis Hypertrophied nails

Onychia Inflammation of nail either post-traumatic or with paronychia

Onychoheterotropia Misplaced nails

Onycholysis Separation of nail from its bed

Onychomadesis Nail shedding starting at base and extending forward (same as defluvium unguium)

Onychomycosis Fungal infection of nail plate

Onychophagia Nail biting

Onychorrhexis Excess longitudinal striation

Onychoschizia Splitting of nails into layers

Onychotillomania Picking at a nail from habit

Pachyonychia Thickening of nail usually increasing from base to tip

Panaritium Abscess at side or base of nail (whitlow)

Paronychia Inflammation of tissues surrounding the nail

Platonychia Increased curvature in long axis

Polyonychia Two or more separate nails on one digit

Pterygium unguis Overgrowth of cuticle on to nail eventually destroying nail

Trachyonychia Rough nails

Unguis incarnatus Ingrowing nail

Usure des ongles Wearing away of nails due to scratching

Appendix II

Relative incidence of nail disorders (1128 patients)

Chronic paronychia	334	Disorders due to impaired circulation	64
Tinea unguium	220	Yellow nail syndrome	21
Abnormalities due to trauma	181	Dermatitis	25
Psoriasis	122	Onycholysis (cause unknown)	46
Miscellaneous acquired nail disorders	66	Developmental anomalies	49

The miscellaneous acquired nail disorders can be further broken down:

Miscellaneous acquired nail disorders (66 patients)

Tumours under or near the nail	15	Candidiasis of nail plates	6
Acute paronychia	11	Acrodermatitis continua	5
Lichen planus	8	Median nail dystrophy	4
		Other conditions	17

INDEX